GROUP TRAUMA TREATMENT
IN EARLY RECOVERY

Also Available

The Trauma Recovery Group:
A Guide for Practitioners

*Michaela Mendelsohn, Judith Lewis Herman,
Emily Schatzow, Melissa Coco, Diya Kallivayalil,
and Jocelyn Levitan*

Group Trauma Treatment in Early Recovery

Promoting Safety and Self-Care

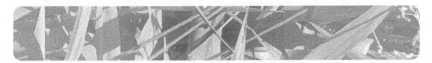

Judith Lewis Herman
Diya Kallivayalil
and Members of the Victims of Violence Program

THE GUILFORD PRESS
New York   London

The authors have checked with sources believed to be reliable in their efforts to provide information
that is complete and generally in accord with the standards of practice that are accepted at the time of
publication. However, in view of the possibility of human error or changes in behavioral, mental health,
or medical sciences, neither the authors, nor the editors and publisher, nor any other party who has been
involved in the preparation or publication of this work warrants that the information contained herein
is in every respect accurate or complete, and they are not responsible for any errors or omissions or the
results obtained from the use of such information. Readers are encouraged to confirm the information
contained in this book with other sources.

Library of Congress Cataloging-in-Publication Data

Names: Herman, Judith Lewis, 1942- author. | Kallivayalil, Diya, author. |
    Victims of Violence Program, issuing body.
Title: Group trauma treatment in early recovery : promoting safety and
    self-care / Judith Lewis Herman, Diya Kallivayalil, and members of the
    Victims of Violence Program
Description: New York : The Guilford Press, [2019] | Includes bibliographical
    references and index.
Identifiers: LCCN 2018012883 | ISBN 9781462537440 (pbk. : alk. paper)
Subjects: | MESH: Psychotherapy, Group—methods | Stress Disorders,
    Post-Traumatic—therapy | Group Processes | Violence—psychology |
    Survivors—psychology | Models, Psychological
Classification: LCC RC510 | NLM WM 430.5 | DDC 616.89/152—dc23
LC record available at *https://lccn.loc.gov/2018012883*

About the Authors

Judith Lewis Herman, MD, is Professor of Psychiatry (part time) at Harvard Medical School. For 30 years, until she retired, she was Director of Training at the Victims of Violence Program (VOV) at Cambridge Health Alliance (CHA) in Cambridge, Massachusetts. She is the author of two award-winning books—*Father–Daughter Incest* and *Trauma and Recovery*—and coauthor of *The Trauma Recovery Group: A Guide for Practitioners*. Dr. Herman is a recipient of the Lifetime Achievement Award from the International Society for Traumatic Stress Studies, the Woman in Science Award from the American Medical Women's Association, and the Lifetime Achievement Award from the Trauma Psychology Division of the American Psychological Association. She is a Distinguished Life Fellow of the American Psychiatric Association.

Diya Kallivayalil, PhD, is a staff psychologist at the VOV Program at CHA and the trauma consultant for the Department of Psychiatry. She is also Assistant Professor in the Department of Psychiatry at Harvard Medical School and a member of the faculty of the CHA's seminar on Global Health and Human Rights. Dr. Kallivayalil's clinical specialty is the treatment of trauma-related disorders. She has published in the areas of complex trauma, gender-based violence, homicide bereavement, and refugee health. She is coauthor of *The Trauma Recovery Group.*

MEMBERS OF THE VICTIMS OF VIOLENCE PROGRAM

Lois Glass, MSW, LICSW, is in private practice and a senior consultant to the VOV Program at CHA. She also is Director of the Vicarious Trauma Project at the Boston Area Rape Crisis Center and a member of the national Vicarious Trauma Toolkit Project, sponsored by the U.S. Department of Justice. Ms. Glass specializes in group treatment and the treatment of trauma. She has lectured extensively and has contributed to many publications, including *Our Bodies, Ourselves.*

Barbara Hamm, PsyD, is a consulting psychologist and Co-Director of Victim Service Initiatives for Violence Transformed at the Public Health Advocacy Institute/Northeastern University School of Law. She is also a licensed clinical psychologist with a private practice and consultation service in Cambridge, Massachusetts, and former Director of the VOV Program at CHA. Dr. Hamm has developed several group therapy models for treating complex trauma, has presented nationally and internationally on the impact of traumatic experiences over the course of the lifespan, has pioneered mindfulness training for law enforcement officers, and has traveled extensively in the United States and abroad to offer trauma training to organizations working with refugees in flight and victims of natural and man-made disasters. She is affiliated with the Center for Mindfulness and Compassion at CHA and is on the technical advisory board for the SEED Foundation in Kurdistan.

Tal Astrachan, PsyD, is a clinical psychologist in private practice in Cambridge and Somerville, Massachusetts. She completed a 2-year postdoctoral fellowship at the VOV Program at CHA, specializing in the assessment and treatment of psychological trauma. She also completed postgraduate training in accelerated experiential dynamic psychotherapy and emotion-focused therapy.

Phillip Murray Brown, MSW, LICSW, is the group coordinator at the VOV Program at CHA, where he offers individual psychotherapy, group psychotherapy, and crisis counseling for survivors of recent violent crime. In addition to his work at the VOV Program, Mr. Brown is Chief of Social Work and Director of Social Work Training for the Department of Psychiatry at CHA, where he also leads a clinical team within general psychiatry as part of the outpatient department. He holds a faculty appointment at Harvard Medical School; is on the adjunct faculty at Tufts University, where he teaches an undergraduate course on sexual assault and domestic violence; and maintains a private practice in Cambridge, Massachusetts.

Preface

HOW THIS BOOK CAME TO BE: A STORY OF GROUP PROCESS

This is a confession of sorts: I feel the need to explain how I came to be the lead author of a treatment guide for a group model that I did not invent, and how my colleagues who did invent the group, and those who have led it in one form or another over the course of many years, have graciously permitted me to take on this role. To explain, I must recount briefly some of the 30-year history of the Victims of Violence (VOV) Program, the home base where this group was developed, practiced, and taught.

When the psychologist Mary Harvey and I cofounded the program in 1984, the Cambridge Hospital Department of Psychiatry, where we were based, was itself a relatively new and creative enterprise. Cambridge Hospital was a public "safety net" hospital with a mission to care for poor people. It was also a teaching hospital for Harvard Medical School. The founders of the psychiatry department were a group of very bright and unconventional young men (yes, all men at the time). They were innovators, interested in expanding the reach of psychiatry into all matters affecting public mental health. When the city of Cambridge appropriated a small sum to the Department of Psychiatry to develop a treatment program for victims of crime, the department chairman was willing to hire two avowed feminists to take on the project. Thus the VOV Program was born.

Small groups had been the organizing tool of the women's liberation movement. According to the theory of consciousness-raising, through sharing personal testimony about the realities of our lives, women could discover the shared truth of our political subordination. Though consciousness-raising groups did not have an avowed therapeutic purpose, nevertheless they owed much of their popularity to the fact that many women found them profoundly therapeutic. The "Aha!" moment of political insight was often inseparable from the moment of personal insight; hence the slogan, "The personal is political."

We knew, therefore, that we wanted to develop groups as one of our treatment offerings, but what kind of groups? There was the model of the "rap groups" of returning war veterans, where men shared the stories of war trauma. Would something similar be useful for crime victims, or would it be too overwhelming for people who had their own private suffering to hear the horrific details of what others had suffered? By contrast, behavioral psychology offered the model of "stress management" groups, which were didactic groups that taught skills like breathing techniques to help deal with traumatic stress symptoms. Would this type of group be more suitable? Learning skills could be helpful, but would victims not feel silenced if they were discouraged from talking about what had happened to them? Thus began an era of experimentation in many forms of group treatment at the VOV Program.

Mary and I wanted to import the wisdom developed in grassroots feminist victim services, like rape crisis centers, into the rarified world of academic psychiatry, which at the time was generally blind to the importance of trauma, and particularly blind to the impact of everyday violence against women. The first staff members we recruited were two social workers from the Boston Area Rape Crisis Center. Both of them are still working at the VOV Program, now among our senior wise women. One of them, Lois Glass, is a coauthor of this book.

We also knew from the outset that teaching and clinical training would be part of the mission of the VOV Program, as it was a basic mission of our teaching hospital. One of our first postdoctoral fellows was a young psychologist, Barbara Hamm. When she completed her training, Barbara joined our growing staff. She has continued at our program throughout her career, eventually becoming the program director when Mary retired. Together, Lois and Barbara originated the Trauma Information Group (TIG).

In the early 1990s, Lois and Barbara were invited to consult at the hospital's psychiatric inpatient service. Though many of the patients had histories of trauma, few were aware of the impact of trauma in their lives. For that matter, the staff, too, seemed unaware, even though by this time a number of studies from around the country had shown that the majority of psychiatric inpatients had significant trauma histories. Inquiring about trauma was not even part of a standard psychiatric history on the inpatient service, and the staff seemed squeamish about making such inquiries.

So Barbara and Lois began to spend time "hanging out" on the inpatient unit, offering to bring patients together for educational group meetings and incidentally educating the staff as well. Many features of the TIG structure were determined initially by the particular conditions of the inpatient service. Each group session had to be relatively self-contained since the membership varied from week to week. The groups had to be carefully structured to make them emotionally tolerable for patients who were at their most vulnerable. And they had to convey some basic information about common reactions to trauma, both in childhood and in adult life.

Starting with just a few topics, Lois wrote a number of educational worksheets for use in the groups. Barbara, whose background was in child psychology, contributed a developmental framework. For each topic, the worksheet began with a description of how a child develops in the context of safe relationships, then moved on to describe the impact of violence and abuse on development. The main point was to normalize traumatic reactions and to place them in a larger social context, so that patients could understand that their traumatic stress symptoms were not a sign of personal defectiveness, but rather a common human response to danger and cruelty.

The group leaders passed around copies of the worksheets and then read them aloud, inviting patients to comment. Reflecting back on that time, Lois reminisced, "You could see the light bulbs going on! Some of these patients had been in psychiatric care for years, but had never had this language to consider before." Soon, patients were suggesting additional topics. "Anger," for example, was not among the original topics. Lois and Barbara attributed this omission to their own female socialization. "We took responsibility for avoiding the topic," says Lois. "We invited the patients to write the worksheet, and they did!" The message, from the outset, was one of respect and empowerment: patients could be collaborators with professionals in the invention of a new form of psychotherapy.

The inpatient service turned out to be a relatively safe setting for figuring out to what degree patients should be encouraged to share the details of their trauma histories. Lois remembered vividly the "scariest moment" in one of the early groups, when a man began a vivid description of how, as an abused child, he had himself tortured animals. "Everyone started dissociating, and the guy apologized and ran out of the room. Barbara ran out after him, and we spent the whole session grounding people. That was the worst." It was from incidents like this one that we determined the main focus of an early-recovery group (what we now call a Stage 1 group) should be on the present rather than on the past.

After pioneering the model on the hospital's inpatient service, Lois and Barbara brought the TIG to the outpatient service where the VOV Program was based. Soon it was among our most popular offerings. By the late 1990s we were running several TIGs each year. The co-leadership model made the group well suited for teaching. After a brief seminar that explained the model, Lois or Barbara would co-lead a group with a trainee, who would then become the "senior" co-leader with a second trainee, and so on. The earliest draft of what became the group manual was written for training purposes at that time.

Over time, Lois took over the basic training for the TIGs offered at the VOV Program. In the past 10 years, Lois has conducted a yearly seminar in which she offers trainees and staff throughout the psychiatry department opportunities to observe her and a trainee co-leading a group. She has steadfastly preserved and taught the TIG model that she originated to many generations of students. Clearly, if not for Lois, there would be no book. In the creation of this book, Lois contributed many clinical illustrations and reflections.

Lois and Barbara have also taught the TIG model at conferences and at many other mental health agencies in the Boston area. The model proved to be highly adaptable for the particular populations served by each agency. One of the first agencies to adopt the model was our sister program, the Boston Area Rape Crisis Center, where Lois eventually became the clinical director. Meanwhile, Barbara has developed many new adaptations of the basic TIG model for the VOV Program, incorporating art, music, and other forms of creativity into her groups. In the writing of this book, Barbara focused on Chapter 6, "Adaptations of the Trauma Information Group."

Phil Brown came to the VOV Program as a social work fellow in 1998 and participated in the "each one teach one" basic training for the TIG. When he finished his training and joined our staff, he soon began to work on adapting our existing group models for male trauma survivors, who constituted about 15% of our patient population. Initially he co-led his male survivor groups with a female staff person. This continued until his co-leader went on vacation, when the group members brought up topics like "intimacy" and "sexuality," which they had been too embarrassed to discuss with a woman present.

Once again, we learned from our patients. From then on, our male survivors' group has had male co-leaders.* Phil remains on the VOV Program staff, where he has now become the coordinator of group services. He has also recently been promoted to the director of social work within CHA's psychiatry department.

Tal Astrachan came to the VOV Program as a psychology postdoctoral fellow a decade after Phil, in 2008–2010. She participated in the basic TIG training, and then co-led two groups with Lois. In fact, she had already had experience with the TIG, for after graduating from college, she had worked for 2 years as a staff member of the Boston Area Rape Crisis Center. "I didn't have very much clinical training, but they let me lead a group with a more experienced staff member, and it was a very positive experience, for me and for the group members," Tal reflected. "I guess if you have genuine respect for the survivors it can come through, even with inexperienced therapists."

While a fellow at the VOV Program, Tal worked on a project to expand the existing TIG manual. One of the groups she co-led with Lois was audiotaped and transcribed. Tal reviewed the transcripts and proposed several basic themes and types of interventions. She, Lois, Barbara, and Phil then coded the transcripts, noting how frequently these themes and interventions appeared. Finally, Tal wrote a draft of a paper about the TIG. Then real life intervened. When Tal completed her fellowship, she took a job in another city and, despite everyone's best intentions, long-distance collaboration proved too difficult. Without Tal's presence, the TIG writing project languished.

In the meantime, however, another of our former psychology postdoctoral fellows, Diya Kallivayalil, had been hired as a staff psychologist by the general outpatient psychiatry department at Cambridge Hospital. During her fellowship at the VOV Program, from 2006 to 2008, Diya had worked with me on a project to create a treatment guide for another of our most successful group models, called the Trauma Recovery Group (TRG). This is a Stage 2, trauma-focused group, a model that I and my colleague Emily Schatzow first developed for incest survivors in the early 1980s. We had then brought it to the VOV Program, where it was adapted for survivors of many kinds of trauma. Diya stayed connected with this writing project, even after her training at the VOV Program ended, and she became one of the coauthors of our book *The Trauma Recovery Group: A Guide for Practitioners*, published by The Guilford Press in 2011.

Once this book was published, the need for a companion volume on the TIG became ever more apparent. Wherever we taught the model for the TRG, it was clear that for every patient who was ready for a Stage 2 group, there were many more who would be better

---

*We don't suggest that this is a general rule. Lois notes that the Boston Area Rape Crisis Center has successfully offered male survivor groups with male and female co-leaders; in fact, some men say they feel safer with female therapists, which makes sense in view of the fact that in most cases their abusers were male.

served by a Stage 1 group like the TIG. I began to hound Lois and Barbara mercilessly about completing the TIG manual for publication, but, realistically, neither one had the time nor the inclination to take the lead. Finally, in exasperation, they declared, "Look, we're not writers. If you really want to get this done, you or someone else will have to do it!"

I talked this situation over with Diya. In 2015, she had taken on responsibility for trauma training in the general outpatient psychiatry department after I retired from my position as training director at the VOV Program. Having already worked together on one book, Diya and I had some experience in bringing the fruits of clinical invention to the written page. We had also coauthored papers, and we knew we enjoyed working together. With my newfound leisure in retirement, I thought that I might be able to take on the responsibility of completing the TIG project, as long as Diya was willing to do it with me. Enthusiastically, she agreed. With Lois and Barbara concurring, Phil and Tal agreed to join in, and our team of authors was complete.

In our writing process, Lois became the voice of TIG experience, channeled throughout the book by Diya, who interviewed her repeatedly and sought her comments on every chapter. Barbara, Phil, and Tal wrote first drafts of Chapters 5 and 6. Diya wrote all the rest. My task was then to revise the entire manuscript, with the goal of preserving, to the best of my ability, the quality of each individual voice, while lending a sense of unity to the whole. Our final product is a guide for a brief (10-session) group treatment that we hope will be suitable for a wide population of trauma survivors in early recovery.

In this brief history, I have tried to capture something of the VOV Program spirit that fostered imagination and creativity and that enabled collaboration across generations. It has been my joy and honor to see the work that Mary and I started half a lifetime ago take hold and flourish. This book is but one of the fruits of the VOV Program. None of us could have written it alone; together we have managed, somehow, to get it done. Another testament, if any were needed, to the power of small groups.

JUDITH LEWIS HERMAN

How to Use This Guide

Leaders of this group should be qualified mental health professionals (e.g., psychologists, social workers, psychiatrists, and psychiatric nurses) with some experience both in working with traumatized clients and in facilitating therapy groups. Students and beginners may co-lead the group with experienced professionals.

Before planning to start a group, we recommend that you read this treatment guide thoroughly from start to finish. You will then be in a position to assess how to adapt it for the patient population that you serve. Chapter 1 reviews the literature on group treatment for interpersonal violence. In Chapters 2–4, we explain how to maintain the educational format of the group while fostering a supportive group process, with concrete, session-by-session instructions. Each of the 10 sessions of the TIG is structured around a worksheet, which is read aloud in the group with pauses for commentary. The worksheets are a versatile tool that may be adapted or translated as needed. They are provided in Appendix C. There is also an online supplement containing Spanish translations of the TIG worksheets from Appendix C. The translations are often useful for clients who are monolingual Spanish, as it gives them an opportunity to use and benefit from the TIG worksheets. They are also an option for a client who is bilingual but whose first language is Spanish. In Chapter 5, we focus on the particular challenges of group leadership. Finally, Chapter 6 provides general guidance on how to adapt the TIG for different populations, with several specific illustrations.

This treatment guide includes many verbatim vignettes from group leaders' interventions, but these are offered as examples only. We strongly advise you not to bring the treatment guide into sessions or to read from it word for word. Our hope is that both new and experienced group leaders will be able to rely on the structure of the group provided here, and that this scaffolding will enable you to use your own voices and styles as you do the powerful work of bearing witness to the trauma of interpersonal violence and to the process of recovery.

How to Use This Guide

Contents

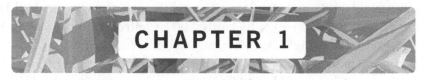

CHAPTER 1

Group Treatment for Interpersonal Violence

In the 26 years since the publication of the classic text *Trauma and Recovery* (Herman, 1992/2015), a collective understanding of the impact of traumatic and violent events—on the brain, on children, on attachment, on health, on society—has expanded. The Adverse Childhood Experiences studies (Felitti et al., 1998) conducted at Kaiser–Permanente and in collaboration with the Centers for Disease Control and Prevention have moved the recognition of the impact of interpersonal trauma out of the cloistered realm of psychiatry into medicine, public health, and the public sphere. Reports from our returning veterans and from college campuses have made us grapple with the pervasiveness of interpersonal violence, while also illuminating the institutional failures that perpetuate it (Armeni, 2014; Sinozich & Langton, 2014).

Trauma and Recovery framed the concept of complex posttraumatic stress disorder (PTSD) as an adaptation to prolonged and repeated abuses, especially those that begin in childhood. Complex PTSD, with its symptom triad of somatization, dissociation, and emotional dysregulation (van der Kolk et al., 1996), is chronic, is often refractory to treatment, and results in significant functional impairment (Courtois & Ford, 2009). The impact of prolonged interpersonal trauma on the lives of its victims is particularly destructive in its social disruption and alienation (Sewell & Williams, 2001). The relational difficulties that plague chronically traumatized people—such as volatile relationships, disordered attachments, and vulnerability to repeated victimization—are well demonstrated in the research (Brown, 2009; Brown, Kallivayalil, & Harvey, 2012; Classen, Palesh, & Aggarwal, 2005; Liotti, 2004). Prolonged trauma simultaneously evokes emotional distress and undermines the capacity to regulate it. Interpersonal violence compromises the victim's access to social support by engendering distrust of others and by shattering assumptions about the safety of the world (Charuvastra & Cloitre, 2008). In addition, the classic symptoms of posttraumatic disorder, such as avoidance and irritability, make it difficult for survivors to build new mutually sustaining relationships (Briere & Rickards, 2007; Cloitre, Miranda, Stovall-McClough, & Han, 2005; van der Kolk, Roth, Pelcovitz, Sunday, & Spinazzola, 2005).

Psychotherapy, a potentially reparative experience, is the treatment of choice for severe and complex trauma (Cloitre et al., 2012). Recovery requires not only the reduction of symptoms, but also an improvement in the capacity for self-regulation and strengthening of interpersonal relationships. While long-term individual psychotherapy is the foundation of treatment, the unequal power dynamics between patient and therapist can create certain limitations. The experience of being subordinated and humiliated by a more powerful person profoundly affects all future relationships, including the therapy relationship. Group therapy, in contrast, can provide survivors of violence an exceptional opportunity to counteract the experience of subordination by joining with peers on a plane of equality to combat social isolation and fear, to relieve shame, to cultivate a sense of belonging, to connect with sources of resilience and self-esteem, and to rebuild the relational capacities shattered by traumatic experience.

There is now considerable evidence that group therapy can also help address an array of posttraumatic symptoms that affect the survivor's sense of self, mood, and daily functioning (e.g., Foy et al., 2000; Shea, McDevitt-Murphy, Ready, & Schnurr, 2009). The importance of group therapy is recognized in the expert consensus guidelines of the International Society for Traumatic Stress Studies (ISTSS). In fact, six of the nine studies cited in the ISTSS best-practice guidelines for complex PTSD used group treatment models (one used group plus individual treatment and another group plus case management; Cloitre et al., 2012).

This treatment guide describes a time-limited approach to group treatment called the Trauma Information Group (TIG). This group model was developed in the early 1990s at the Victims of Violence (VOV) Program, a hospital-based outpatient program serving survivors of complex trauma at Cambridge Health Alliance. Since that time, over 60 groups have been conducted, with more than 500 trauma survivors. In studies conducted at our clinic, most participants in the TIG made significant improvements in measures of depression, posttraumatic stress, dissociation, and self-esteem (Mendelsohn et al., 2011).

The TIG model has also been used in multiple other treatment settings. It has proved to be a very durable and adaptable group model for trauma survivors in an early stage of recovery. The group is unique in that it *combines a grounding, psychoeducational, and cognitive framework with a carefully constructed supportive relational group process* that is particularly well suited to early-stage trauma treatment. Like some other group models, it utilizes educational worksheets that provide information about trauma and recovery to structure the group and homework handouts to help patients deepen their understanding of trauma and build new coping skills. Unlike other existing models, however, the TIG manual also includes specific instructions for group leaders on how to build on the unique therapeutic potential of a group by developing an interpersonal process that relieves shame and fosters a sense of belonging. For these reasons, we believe that this treatment guide for the TIG will constitute an original and useful contribution to the field and a unique, accessible, and adaptable model for trauma clinicians in a multitude of settings.

THE TRAUMA INFORMATION GROUP

The conceptual framework for this group is derived from the stage model of treatment for complex trauma outlined in *Trauma and Recovery* (Herman, 1992/2015). The stage model, a widely accepted and adopted metamodel of trauma treatment, is recommended by the expert consensus guidelines of the ISTSS (Cloitre et al., 2012). In contrast with trauma treatments that begin at once to focus on telling the trauma story, in a staged model of recovery, the initial focus of treatment in the *first stage* of recovery involves the establishment of *safety*. Both individual and group treatment interventions at this stage are focused on symptom mastery, stabilization, and the basic routines of self-care. Therapy focuses on the body (establishing daily rhythms of sleeping and eating, managing intrusive PTSD symptoms, and reducing self-harming behaviors), on the environment (establishing a secure living situation and having steady work and financial stability), and on safe interpersonal relations (building a trustworthy social support system with mutual, nonexploitative relationships). This early stage of treatment is often the most demanding and prolonged.

The rationale for a staged model of recovery is that without establishing safety in the present, exploration of the traumatic past simply becomes another experience of trauma. Once safety is established in the present, it becomes possible for the survivor to revisit the horrors of the past, rather than simply to relive them. The therapeutic task of the *second stage* of treatment involves a carefully paced, in-depth *exploration and processing* of the traumatic memories so that they can be integrated into a coherent and nuanced life narrative. Once this stage is completed, it becomes possible for the survivor to envision a future, and preoccupation with the past gives way naturally to a focus on rebuilding a life. The *third stage* of recovery therefore involves *reconnecting* with the survivor's larger community (Herman, 1992/2015).

Stage 1 groups are designed to meet the goals of safety, stability, and self-care. They are present focused, they generally have a didactic component, and they usually discourage detailed trauma disclosure to prevent group members from becoming overwhelmed (Harney & Harvey, 1999). The TIG is conceptualized as a Stage 1 group. Its tasks include increasing the capacity for modulating extreme arousal states, reducing trauma-related avoidance, deepening understanding of the impact of trauma, and developing both a sense of basic agency and a sense of peer support (Courtois, Ford, & Cloitre, 2009). The focus of the TIG on early recovery issues; its relatively brief time frame (usually 10–14 sessions); and its combination of a structured, educational, and cognitive framework and a supportive, relational group process make it well suited as a "beginners" group for patients who have only recently started treatment.

Though the combination of individual and group therapy is often highly effective, we have found that individual therapy is not a necessary prerequisite for this group. Over the years, the TIG has been adapted for use in many different settings, including an inpatient unit, a gay and lesbian counseling program, a rape crisis center, and a Latino mental health program where worksheets were translated into Spanish and modified to include the impact of political trauma and issues of acculturation. Most recently, the TIG has been adapted for rural Native Canadian trauma survivors, for mostly undocumented immigrant workers who retrieved the remains of the dead from Ground Zero, and for women with HIV/AIDS, many of whom have histories of severe trauma. The worksheets can be expanded or shortened, and clinicians can develop additional worksheets for the populations they serve (see Chapter 6).

The TIG is designed for patients who may have little understanding of how traumatic events have affected their lives. Survivors who are just beginning to explore the relationship between their traumatic past and their current life patterns are appropriate candidates for this group, as are those whose lives are marked by social isolation. Many patients who participate in this group have never spoken about their traumatic experiences to anyone or have shared it only with significant others who have minimized, denied, or invalidated the significance of the trauma. This group, for many, is their first experience meeting others who recognize that the trauma has had a significant and harmful impact and who understand that they are not responsible for the abuse they suffered.

The TIG has a deceptively simple structure, which in practice serves multiple complex functions. Many Stage 1 group treatments have a cognitive and psychoeducation orientation, as the TIG does; however, in the TIG the *interpersonal* or relational nature of the group context ("the groupness of the group") is emphasized; it is not simply a class on trauma and recovery, nor is it cognitive-behavioral therapy done in a group context. Patients are encouraged to share the relational impact of trauma, and this kind of sharing allows them to develop a sense of belonging and to be relieved of shame. The structure is designed to facilitate interpersonal exchange, while minimizing disclosure and maximizing affiliation and mastery. In this way, the group provides an opportunity to begin the recovery process while adhering to the principle of safety.

Each group usually contains 6 to 10 members and ideally should be co-led by two therapists. The usual length of group sessions is 10–14 weeks. Each group session usually lasts 1 hour. The treatment model lends itself to this relatively short group session, as it is designed to be containing rather than exploratory. The structure of the group is discussed in greater detail in Chapter 2. Modifications of the usual structure are reviewed in Chapter 6.

Each group session focuses on a topic related to the impact of trauma; examples include Safety and Self-Care, Trust, Anger, Remembering, and Shame. Topical worksheets help group members to develop a cognitive framework for understanding the impact of trauma on their current lives. Each week the worksheets build on each other, starting with the topics that most easily facilitate bonding and progressing to more challenging topics.

Most of the patients seen at the VOV Program are survivors of childhood trauma. Therefore, our standard worksheets begin by explaining what would be the optimal developmental process for children in a safe and supportive environment. They then go on to describe how childhood trauma can affect this process. Each worksheet outlines the many emotional, cognitive, and behavioral ways trauma survivors cope that may have been adaptive at the time, but that may cause considerable suffering later on. For example, in the Trust session, a number of people might share how from a very early age they learned not to trust. Someone might share a story of how she assumed throughout her life that people were going to hurt her and how she never let anyone in. She may then discuss her contemporary struggles in the trust arena and connect the past and present, leading group members to reflect on how hard it is to let go of the past.

The worksheets are read aloud in the group, one or two paragraphs at a time, and members comment on them and share relevant stories from their own life experiences. Group leaders model empathic feedback and encourage group members to offer compassion and understanding to one another. Group members frequently comment on how relieving this framework is because it makes many of the experiences they find particularly distressing comprehensible to them as consequences of trauma, rather than as a sign of personal defectiveness.

The focus of the group on the *impact* of trauma, rather than on details of the trauma history, helps members titrate and regulate affect, so as to make addressing trauma-related issues manageable. It also provides an experience in which group members can learn to reference and discuss their trauma histories without disclosing every detail in an unmodulated way. This in itself is often a vastly important interpersonal skill for survivors, who may feel that their only options are either to hide their trauma histories from others or to disclose indiscriminately.

By witnessing both the struggles and the strengths of other trauma survivors, group members often come to feel markedly less alone. Discovering that they can be helpful to others, group members develop a sense of competence and pride. In offering compassion and empathy to others, group members are often enabled to develop increased compassion and empathy for themselves.

THE "EVIDENCE BASE"

Outcome research generally supports group therapy for patients with PTSD, but does not favor one type of group over another. Foy and colleagues (2000), who conducted a comprehensive review of empirical studies, found that group psychotherapy was associated with positive outcomes in a range of symptoms, regardless of treatment approach or model; improvements in PTSD symptoms, dissociation, global distress, and self-esteem were all noted. More recently, Fritch and Lynch (2008), in a similar review, found that many studies reported improvement on measures of interpersonal functioning, as well as symptom reduction. The range of group treatment approaches included affect management (Zlotnick et al., 1997), dialectical behavior therapy (DBT) skills plus writing-based exposure (Bradley & Follingstad, 2003), psychoeducation (Lubin, Loris, Burt, & Johnson, 1998), cognitive processing therapy (Chard, 2005), trauma-focused therapy (Classen, Koopman, Nevill-Manning, & Spiegel, 2001), interpersonal therapy (Cloitre & Koenen, 2001; Ray & Webster, 2010), and process groups (Hazzard, Rogers, & Angert, 1993).

There is no evidence supporting the superiority of one group model of treatment over another (Sloan, Feinstein, Gallagher, Beck, & Keane, 2013). In fact, very few studies have directly compared the effectiveness of two different types of group therapy for interpersonal trauma survivors. Dunn and colleagues (2007) compared the efficacy of a self-management group versus psychoeducation for a cohort of veterans with comorbid PTSD and depression. The self-management intervention appeared to show initial gains for depression symptoms, but this difference did not persist at follow-up. A randomized controlled study by Classen and colleagues (2001) with adult female childhood sexual abuse survivors assigned participants to either trauma-focused group therapy, person-centered group therapy, or a wait-list group. Participants in both treatment conditions showed significant improvement on trauma-related symptoms, while the wait-list controls did not. Finally, 360 male veterans with chronic combat-related PTSD were randomly assigned to trauma-focused or person-centered group therapy for 25 weekly therapy sessions (Schnurr et al., 2003). PTSD and other symptoms were significantly improved for both conditions, but there were no overall differences between the two types of group therapy on any outcome measure.

We wonder whether it would have been possible to discriminate between the effectiveness of these two types of group therapy if the authors of these randomized controlled trials had taken account of the stages of recovery. We suspect that patients in Stage 1 would have done better in the person-centered group, while patients who were ready for Stage 2 work would have done better in the trauma-focused group. It is worth noting that treatment dropout was higher among those assigned to the trauma-focused group. This outcome is just what one would expect if patients in early recovery were assigned to a type of group for which they were not ready.

Comparable Group Manuals

Very few group models for trauma survivors in early recovery have been developed into published treatment manuals. With one exception, existing manuals are designed either for individual or for group psychotherapy, with little if any discussion of either the potential power or the particular demands of group treatment. The three that most closely resemble the TIG are called Trauma Recovery and Empowerment (TREM), Seeking Safety (SS), and Trauma-Centered Group Psychotherapy (TCGP). The TREM model (Fallot & Harris, 2002; Harris, 1998) was originally designed to serve impoverished women with histories of childhood abuse living with the cumulative effects of poverty and stigma. It is based on the principles of cognitive restructuring, skills development, and psychoeducation and has three major sections: empowerment for women, trauma education, and skills building. The group model has been implemented in a wide range of agencies, including residential and nonresidential substance abuse and mental health programs, correctional facilities, health clinics, and welfare-to-work programs, among others, particularly in urban areas. Twenty-four to 29 topics are covered in weekly 75-minute meetings; each topic is introduced with a brief clinical rationale, a set of goals, questions to be posed to the group, and an experiential exercise. An adaptation for Latina women has been developed and published in a separate manual. One outcome study has shown promising results for reducing trauma symptoms, improving coping, and reducing general substance abuse (Fallot, McHugo, Harris, & Xie, 2011); another study showed that women who participated in TREM had significantly better outcomes for trauma-related symptoms than those who received treatment as usual, but better outcomes were not found for alcohol or drug use.

The SS model was developed by Najavits (2002) for clients with dual diagnoses of PTSD and substance abuse. It is conceptualized as a cognitive-behavioral treatment with influences from 12-step programs and other self-help traditions. SS does not include discussion of specific trauma memories and is best conceptualized as a Stage 1 treatment. It can be offered as either an individual or a group treatment. Twenty-five topics are discussed, and clients are asked to identify a safe coping skill. More than 80 "safe coping" skills are taught in a curriculum that has defined topics and structured exercises. Various studies have shown the effectiveness of SS in reducing PTSD and substance abuse (Desai, Harpaz-Rotem, Najavits, & Rosenheck, 2008; Hien, Cohen, Miele, Litt, & Capstick, 2004; Najavits, Weiss, Shaw, & Muenz, 1998). A recent summary of the evidence, however, argues that SS is not superior to other active treatments, such as psychoeducation (Sloan & Beck, 2016).

TCGP (Lubin & Johnson, 2008) was created specifically to address the interpersonal effects of psychological trauma. The group has both a didactic component and an exposure element and therefore is somewhat of a hybrid between a Stage 1 and Stage 2 group. There are 16 weekly sessions, with a lecture topic, handouts and homework assignments, and a "graduation ceremony" at the end of the group. The group was originally developed for women, but it has since been adapted for men, veterans, and women with concurrent PTSD and substance abuse. A nonrandomized outcome study showed that the model is effective in reducing PTSD and depression symptoms, and gains were maintained at a 6-month follow-up (Lubin et al., 1998), but we could not find more recent studies of this treatment method.

Other manualized therapies are comparable to some degree. The most well known, DBT, is a cognitive-behavioral treatment consisting of behavioral skills training originally developed for chronically suicidal individuals with borderline personality disorder, which is now used for a wide range of disorders in which emotional dysregulation is a core feature (see Lynch, Trost, Salsman, & Linehan, 2007, for a review; Salsman & Linehan, 2006). Given the high prevalence of childhood abuse among individuals with borderline personality disorder (upward of 75% have experienced childhood abuse [Herman, Perry, & van der Kolk, 1989; Zanarini, Williams, Lewis, & Reich, 1997] and up to 90% have experienced adult trauma [Zanarini, Frankenburg, Reich, Hennen, & Silk, 2005]), DBT groups are frequently used with trauma survivors, even though there is no explicit recognition of the impact of trauma in the model. The behavioral analysis and skills work that are the cornerstones of DBT can be helpful in addressing the various deficits in self-care and self-soothing that are features of complex traumatic stress disorders. There is a growing attempt to integrate and build a bridge to complex trauma applications among DBT scholars and practitioners (Harned & Linehan, 2008; Swenson, 2000; Wagner, Rizvi, & Harned, 2007). DBT can be implemented in either an individual or group format or with a combination of the two.

TARGET (Ford & Russo, 2006) is another cognitive-behavioral treatment designed to enhance affect regulation without trauma memory processing. It provides psychoeducation that explains PTSD symptoms and affect dysregulation as the results of biological adaptations to survive trauma. Like all the other models we have discussed (with the one exception of TCGP), TARGET can be offered either individually or in a group setting. Restoring affect regulation is described as requiring seven practical steps, or skills, summarized by the acronym "FREEDOM" (where F = Focus the mind on one thought at a time, R = Recognize specific stress triggers, E = Emotion self-check and Evaluate thoughts, D = Define goals, O = Options, and M = Make a contribution). Each chapter of TARGET describes the key points of the lesson, teaching examples, session scripts, and activities, and it can be offered in 12 weeks or adapted for longer treatment trajectories. Studies have shown promise for the TARGET treatment model in various settings in both individual and group therapy contexts (Ford, Steinberg, & Zhang, 2011; Frisman, Ford, Lin, Mallon, & Chang, 2008).

Special Features of the Trauma Information Group

The TIG has a number of features in common with the manualized models described previously; it was originally developed mainly for women survivors of childhood abuse and has since been adapted for many other populations, it is time limited, and it is most appropriate for survivors in early recovery. It uses a didactic format with weekly topics and worksheets. However, it also differs from these models in a number of ways. As compared to SS and TREM, the TIG has a shorter time frame (10–14 weeks), in part to make the group tolerable to members so early in recovery. A shorter time frame also makes groups relatively easy to implement and to offer frequently.

TIG also explicitly draws on the therapeutic action of the group context. Caring interaction and witnessing among group members are powerful mechanisms for normalizing traumatic experience, reducing shame and isolation, and building self-compassion. The TIG manual offers group leaders specific instructions on how to manage potentially disruptive interactions among group members and how to model empathic but containing feedback. Surprisingly, the other existing manuals offer little direction on how to foster a therapeutic interpersonal climate. For those manualized treatments that can be offered either in a group or individually, little attention is given to the ways in which group therapy differs from individual therapy. The therapeutic potential of the bonds that develop between group members is not discussed. By contrast, the TIG manual contains clear instructions for group leaders to maximize the power of this therapeutic modality.

A note about the pronouns used in this treatment guide: Our collective experience with implementing this group treatment approach has primarily been with women survivors of interpersonal trauma. Therefore, this book is based on a women's group, and female pronouns are used to refer to group members and leaders. However, as is discussed in Chapters 2, 4, and 6, the TIG model has also been successfully applied in mixed-gender and men's groups and on occasion with transgender clients.

An additional note about the clinical examples in the book: The clinical material includes case descriptions and modified transcripts from actual clients, as well as composite examples based on the notes of group leaders. We have changed demographic information and other identifying details to preserve anonymity. All the names used are pseudonyms. Clients who participated in the observation groups consented to having their sessions observed.

CONCLUSION

We believe this versatile group model will be suitable for many different populations, as it has already been adapted and used in various settings and with a wide range of patients. The worksheets alone can serve as a comprehensive educational tool, summarizing basic knowledge on many aspects of trauma and trauma recovery. They can be a useful guide to the many aspects of recovery for patients and therapists alike. The group has utility and practicality in numerous clinical settings. The manual has specific instructions about how to run the group, attend to problems, and screen patients, directly addressing the training that therapists need to facilitate the group successfully. The model is unique in that it understands complex PTSD as the consequence of relational harm that needs to be repaired in a relational manner. As an early recovery group that is both educational and relational, we believe the TIG has stood the test of time.

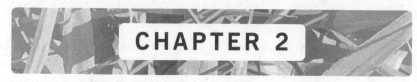

CHAPTER 2

Overview of
the Trauma Information Group

In keeping with its design as a Stage 1 group, the TIG's overriding purpose is to provide a safe environment that allows members to connect with one another and to begin becoming empowered with regard to the impact of traumatic experience on their lives, while adhering to the principles of safety and stabilization.

Many survivors come to the group with a history of having hidden important aspects of themselves, often related to their history of trauma. They talk about showing a "social face" but not letting other people see beneath this surface. A group may provide their first opportunity to be authentic and to connect with others who share similar experiences.

Trauma survivors often function on the extremes of a disclosure continuum. On the one hand, they may sometimes feel pressured to talk in detail about their history, overwhelming themselves and often frightening others. At the other extreme, they may completely isolate themselves, sharing nothing with anyone. This can significantly affect their engagement in the world, making the group possibly the only environment in which they come into contact with other people in anything but a cursory manner. This group offers survivors the opportunity to understand how past trauma affects them today *and* to learn how to communicate this understanding to others. Issues such as how and when to disclose, how much to disclose, and to whom to disclose are all addressed. Members are also encouraged to think realistically about the ways in which their disclosure affects others. Many survivors live with such anxiety and self-consciousness that they do not always consider their impact on others or, if they do, they may have distorted and catastrophic fantasies about how others will respond.

Leaders and other group members help model strategies about disclosure. From the start, leaders discuss how challenging it can be to connect to others and how it takes time to feel safe and to be known in the group. They highlight the impact of disclosures: that they can be overwhelming to hear and also possibly overexposing to the speaker. They encourage sharing that is paced and measured. One member who repeated the group commented to new group members during the start of the first session that this aspect felt the most important to her, letting her consider other ways to be real, while also "testing the waters." She said, "I tell people a little now when I meet them and then choose how and when to say more."

By definition, survivors of interpersonal trauma have experienced relationships characterized by the imposition of power. They are often expert in the nuances of unequal power hierarchies. It is often a new experience for survivors to be exposed to a model of leadership wherein power is shared equally and with mutual respect. For this reason, group leaders need to be conscious of the way in which they share responsibilities and manage their relationship. Leaders do not have to be equal in terms of seniority or professional status. For example, at the VOV Program, where groups are usually co-led by a staff member and a trainee, a power differential between leaders clearly exists. What is important is that leaders acknowledge and recognize this power differential and treat each other respectfully.

A second level of fostering respectful egalitarian relationships occurs through the group structure. Constructive exchange between members, which includes respect and appreciation for differences, is encouraged. Many trauma survivors grew up in environments where differences were punished. A curiosity and respect for how people have coped differently with abuse is a theme of this group. For example, in the Body Image session of the group, members may discuss how some of them have coped by hiding their bodies behind large clothing, while others may point to how they exercise obsessively.

The TIG model is based on the belief that "knowledge is power." Many trauma survivors do not fully understand how their present distress connects with their histories. Helping survivors gain a fuller knowledge of themselves and how their history impacts their current functioning is one of the most important lessons of the group. Hence, "The Impact of Trauma: Posttraumatic Stress Reactions" is the first topic because it provides an organizing conceptual framework.

Group members are also fully informed about the structure and content of the group. At the first group meeting, members are given a list of topics that the group will cover each week (see Appendix A). This concrete information demystifies the group and makes the sessions more predictable. Mastery comes from predictability. In our experience, the more predictable a session can be, the less anxiety it provokes.

Information flows not only from the group leaders but also from the group members to one another. All have stories about how they have coped with trauma that are of great value to others. Survivors often do not appreciate their own resilience or strength and may feel that they do not have anything to offer. Our view is that all survivors must be resilient in some way to have made it thus far. Group members begin to see their own resilience and strength through helping others. They begin to recognize how they have adapted and survived. Measured sharing about successful coping is encouraged in this group.

Group members who also have a relationship with an individual therapist are encouraged to talk about their experience of the group in their therapy. In addition to the worksheets that are discussed in each group session (see Appendix B), members are given optional homework with questions that they can address outside the group therapy session. They are encouraged to bring the worksheets and the homework questions to the individual therapy session. This is not a requirement for the group, but for some it creates an anchor that facilitates continued dialogue. The group leaders do not generally inquire about this process, in part to respect the boundaries the group works to create, and also because leaders do not want people to feel defective if they have not done their homework.

Many group members over the years have said that they have never seen information about trauma exposure and recovery covered as cogently as they have seen it in our handouts and worksheets. Through the information presented in the handouts and worksheets, survivors are encouraged to take an active role in their own recovery. Furthermore, clients are encouraged to learn to pay attention to and honor their comfort level with regard to participation in the group. For example, a client is welcome to state that she does not want to answer a question if she feels overwhelmed in the moment.

GENERAL GOALS

As reflected in the group worksheets, the TIG addresses many interrelated developmental tasks that are derailed in the context of trauma. The TIG includes the following major goals.

1. Increased understanding of the impact of trauma.
2. Decreased sense of isolation and aloneness.
3. Reduced sense of shame, self-blame, and defectiveness.
4. Increased capacity for self-compassion.
5. Increased ability to titrate and regulate trauma-related affect.
6. Enhanced coping skills.
7. Increased capacity for safe relationships.
8. Increased sense of mastery and empowerment.

Interventions are organized around meeting these goals, as well as addressing individual and group processes that may disrupt work toward these goals. We use examples of dialogue that are adapted from transcripts of group sessions to illustrate these points.

Increased Understanding of the Impact of Trauma

Psychoeducation about the impact of trauma on various aspects of development and the self is the foundation of this group. The worksheets anchor the group in an ongoing effort to deepen the group's understanding of the impact of trauma. Often, the simple fact that the worksheets are tangible written documents that externally reflect the experiences of group members *and* relate those experiences to the impact of trauma is experienced as a revelation by group members. Members often make comments such as "You must be psychic" or "It feels like you wrote this thinking about me, even though you don't know me" or "This is really hitting the mark." Sharing worksheets can also lead to a deeper feeling of connection among group members, as people read the material and feel understood. In a recent group, a member said, "To read on paper what we've already talked about in the group, it makes me realize, wow, it's not just me! A lot of people struggle with the same stuff." The topics themselves, each discussed in detail, with information about optimal development and how trauma can disrupt it, can deepen an understanding of the complex and interrelated effects of trauma.

Group leaders ask the members basic questions to begin discussion of the topics. For example, after reading a paragraph of a worksheet out loud, the leaders might ask which sentence of the paragraph that was just read group members can relate to, and why. It is important to avoid asking yes and no questions because it is helpful for group members to have a structure that allows them to articulate their experiences more clearly. Group leaders also frequently offer psychoeducational comments about the impact of trauma and the process of healing throughout group sessions, as relevant to the discussion. Directions about how to foster these discussions are provided in Chapters 3 and 4.

An example of an effective use of psychoeducation is a group session that addresses Body Image. As members read through the worksheet, group leaders often comment on how issues related to body image extend beyond trauma survivors. They can attempt to foster a discussion about how survivors of interpersonal violence think of themselves as fundamentally more damaged than others, and it can be a new experience for them to recognize that their distress is also part of a more universal phenomenon. It can be helpful for group members to realize that most, if not all, women feel negatively about their bodies.

Reduced Isolation and Sense of Aloneness

Social isolation and an overwhelming sense of being alone are among the hallmarks of interpersonal trauma. Over time, enduring feelings of shame and otherness can lead to almost complete social withdrawal or to very limited interpersonal relationships that have constrained dynamics (e.g., becoming the caretaker to an aging perpetrating parent). Connecting with other group members who have had similar difficulties is a powerful vehicle for combating these feelings of isolation and can lay a foundation for enabling the survivor to connect with others in their lives outside the group. Often, merely sitting for the first time in a room with other trauma survivors goes a long way toward addressing this goal. Group members frequently comment that they have never spoken before with someone who has had experiences similar to theirs, or that they are surprised at how "normal" the other group members look.

When a group member indicates a belief that her or his symptoms, feelings, or behavior are particularly unusual or embarrassing, the leaders will ask how many other group members have had similar feelings. Leaders ask for a show of hands and then encourage group members to look around and register their connections. Many trauma survivors spent much of their childhoods not looking directly at their abusive parents, and this avoidance of eye contact can be a barrier to intimacy when it persists into adulthood. The group leaders' interventions directly challenge this avoidant behavior. Group leaders can also intervene to connect seemingly disparate behaviors of group members by highlighting how they are different ways of dealing with the same problem. For example, one group member may avoid intimacy by having numerous fleeting and impersonal sexualized relationships so that she can feel in control of the situation. Another group member may deal with the same fears by avoiding any sexual situation altogether. The group does not process interactions between members, but group leaders regularly ask members to reflect on their commonalities, as in the following example:

GROUP LEADER: What is it like sitting here, listening to other members?

GROUP MEMBER 1: I think [group member 2] is so brave for what she just said.

GROUP LEADER: Do you ever feel that way about yourself?

GROUP MEMBER 1: Never

OTHER MEMBERS: (*Nod collectively, some of them murmuring, "I really get that."*)

Another example of how group leaders work to address isolation and find commonality comes from the session on anger.

GROUP MEMBER 1: I'm one of those people that never gets angry about anything, but I wasn't always that way. I experienced a lot of retaliation for my anger, so I just learned to put it in a box and ignore it. So I know it's in there somewhere but it's not something I want to get into; I don't know if I could handle that.

GROUP LEADER: I just want to point out that intellectual understanding is an important part of feeling more in control of your anger and learning that you can handle it. Maybe something about that allows just an inch of room to be angry about how you've been treated. It's not an all-or-nothing thing.

Notice that the group leader normalizes and reframes this group member's experience, so that expressing feelings of anger do not isolate or stigmatize her within the group. The group then continues.

GROUP MEMBER 2: I feel really angry at being silenced so many years ago, to the point where I developed all kinds of messed-up ways of treating myself. I feel furious about that lost time and how crazy my life got.

GROUP LEADER: Who else in the room has feelings like that? (*Group members all raise their hands.*) That is not an uncommon experience at all—anger and grief about what has gone on.

GROUP MEMBER 2: How do you deal with that?

GROUP LEADER: Just what you're doing, talking about it. It doesn't make it like it never happened, but at least you don't feel so alone with it.

GROUP MEMBER 2: I really do feel alone.

GROUP LEADER: But you also saw everyone in this room raise their hands.

GROUP MEMBER 2: That made me feel a lot better, I have to say.

Reduction in Shame, Self-Blame, and a Sense of Defectiveness

Shame is among the most enduring effects of chronic interpersonal trauma. The literature is rife with studies of trauma survivors who describe their self-image as one of fundamental brokenness. This defective self-image is accompanied by intense feelings of self-disgust and self-hatred (Fonagy, Target, Gergely, Allen, & Bateman, 2003). Participation in a group of fellow survivors, slowly making oneself known in a safe and structured setting, and realizing one's commonalities can provide a powerful antidote to shame and stigma.

The group addresses this issue directly by devoting an entire session to the topic of Shame and Self-Blame. In addition, the various interventions in the TIG associated with decreasing isolation are also aimed at helping group members to reduce their shame, self-blame, and sense of defectiveness. The worksheets help to explain many of the behaviors that survivors feel most ashamed of, such as substance abuse or self-injury, as attempts to manage the emotional impact of trauma. Group leaders initiate and encourage reflection about the origin of these behaviors as efforts to cope, within the limitations of a frequently terrifying and neglectful environment. This discussion allows group members to begin to make sense of their behaviors, even if these behaviors are now no longer adaptive. Group members are frequently able to help other members understand this idea, such that they both can feel that they have something to offer one another. Explaining to others also helps group members deepen their understanding of themselves. Receiving compassion and acceptance from the other group members slowly begins to shift each survivor's defiled sense of self.

The following dialogue is an example from a session on shame.

GROUP LEADER 1: Why else do people feel ashamed of the abuse they experience?

GROUP MEMBER 1: Some kinds of abuse, like with sexual abuse, go with some kind of neglect. So if I turn up to school not dressed right for the weather and my clothes are really old, my parents are the ones who should be ashamed about that, but I am the one who is there. And so you get judgment from teachers and peers about it.

GROUP LEADER 1: So [group member 1] is bringing up another important point, that the child is often too young to realize that it isn't her fault. You come to school and you look disheveled, and you're the one standing there, as you so rightly put it.

GROUP MEMBER 2: Sometimes the abuser tells you that it's your fault.

GROUP LEADER 1: Absolutely. How many people in here have been told by an abuser that it's their fault? So look at that, almost everyone in the room. What does hearing that do to a child or an adult who is vulnerable?

GROUP MEMBER 3: It makes you feel really guilty and like maybe it really is your fault or you asked for it.

GROUP MEMBER 1: For me, I wind up doing this thing now as an adult, where if I do anything wrong, I wind up feeling like I have to mentally punish myself, withdraw, like the worksheet says. And I almost grovel, like, I'm sorry, I'll do better next time.

GROUP LEADER 2: Can people relate to that? Like if you make a regular kind of mistake, like a day-to-day thing like forgetting something?

GROUP MEMBER 4: Yeah, I get preoccupied with how the other person is thinking or feeling toward me if I made a mistake, and I can be terrified way beyond what makes sense.

GROUP LEADER 1: Why are survivors often worried about what other people are thinking?

GROUP MEMBER 5: Because they expect they're going to get hurt. They expect that if they make the other person angry, he's going to hurt you or take something away from you.

GROUP LEADER 1: Let's see if we can get to the people who haven't had a chance to say much today. [Group member 6], is there anything [group member 5] is saying that you can relate to?

GROUP MEMBER 6: I can relate to what you're saying about things you do in certain situations. Like, I can't believe I'm saying this, I used to show up in school kind of unclean and my hair in knots, and you can't understand how it reflects on anybody other than you, especially when you're surrounded by peers who find you repulsive. So the only conclusion you can come to is that you're garbage.

GROUP LEADER 2: Absolutely. And from where you are at now, can you come to another conclusion?

GROUP MEMBER 6: I'm trying to.

GROUP LEADER 1: Sometimes it's easier to feel shame than to feel fear or fury at the people who should have taken care of you and didn't. Sometimes shame can feel emotionally safer in some way. Does that make sense to people?

As another example, in a recent group on Shame and Self-Blame, one of the group members, Maria, started crying as another member was taking her turn toward the end of the group. She said that she felt like a failure compared to the other women in the group because her impression was that they all fought back against their perpetrators while she did not. She shared that when she was raped in college by her boyfriend, she did not "fight back," in part because she was too intoxicated, but primarily because she was so stunned and in disbelief about what was happening. Hearing some of the details of other survivors' stories in the group week after week had made her feel some old, deeply held feelings of guilt, shame, and self-blame. Her impression was that if she had only physically fought back, she might have escaped. "I still feel like a coward today," she said.

Another group member responded, "I understand where you are coming from, but I really disagree with how you are framing what happened to you. From where I sit, you did the best you could in the moment, and whatever you did, or in this case didn't do, it was the right thing because it allowed you to survive the attack and go on to live a life. You could have been even more badly injured than you were if you had fought back and maybe would not be here in this group to talk about it."

Another member chimed in at this point and said that she too has lived with guilt and shame and self-blame most of her life: "I didn't fight back against my abuser either because it was my father, and I knew deep inside that my mother would not believe me and I would be told it was my fault." She went on to recount that a previous therapist helped her have compassion for the girl that she was, and she was able to move to a place of less judgment and more compassion for herself. She said, "Whenever I see a group of middle school or high school girls, I am struck by how young they really are, how they are really just children, in fact." She said that she tries to have empathy for the child she was and appreciate how little power she had to stop what was happening to her in a family where violence was so pervasive.

Maria cried harder in response to these words and said that she so appreciated how kind the other group members were being to her. The group leader responded by suggesting that Maria take with her as much as she could of the other members' compassion and understanding, and her hope was that she would allow that self-compassion to become integrated into her own story, so that it would take up more space over time, as her guilt and self-blame receded.

Increased Capacity for Self-Compassion

This goal is closely related to the previous goal of reducing shame. Group members frequently feel very connected to and compassionate toward other group members. This dynamic allows for interventions unique to a group format that can help members develop compassion for themselves over time. When group leaders notice that a group member is being particularly self-critical or expressing a distorted view of herself, they can ask a question like, "If someone else in the group said that about herself, what would you say?" Members can often recognize that they would offer quite a compassionate response to other group members, and they are encouraged to begin to practice offering themselves a similarly compassionate response. This can be seen as an exercise in mentalization, keeping their own "mind in mind" and recognizing their unconscious distorted self-judgments, particularly in interpersonal situations (Bateman & Fonagy, 2004; Fonagy & Target, 2002). They are also encouraged to keep the other person's mind in mind, and are asked to expand their views of what other people may be feeling and thinking, with direct feedback in the group setting. Over time, this approach can alter the pathologically negative relationship with the self with which many survivors of complex trauma struggle. Group leaders also often explicitly intervene to reinforce and praise the efforts of group members and to encourage them to take credit for successes.

This is an example of a group interaction from the closing round of the session on shame.

> GROUP MEMBER: I'm kind of mixed up. It's hard because I look around and feel so much respect for everyone in here and I identify with so much of it, it's really stupid that I have so much shame about myself. I mean, it just seems illogical.
>
> GROUP LEADER: You know, one of the first steps in dealing with illogical shame can be participating in a group like this and realizing if everyone else deserves a break, maybe you do too.

The following clinical vignette from a TIG with all-male membership also illustrates the power of the group to increase self-compassion for trauma survivors. One of the members, Sean, described living with his father who had abused him as a child, and said that he had been unable to pass the nursing boards, after trying multiple times, so he could get a job and move out. "I hate living with my father," he said, "but I stay there out of fear and because I still feel that I can't support myself." In the group on Anger, Sean described sometimes "shaking with rage" in his room after another verbal altercation with his father, in which his father once again shamed him saying, "If it weren't for me you would be living on the streets. You are nothing without me. You need me." The group tried to encourage Sean to shift his perspective to a point where his father's financial support came with too high a cost.

In the following group session on Relationships, Sean said that although he had appreciated the group's support the previous week, it felt like too much of a risk to go out on his own now because every time he had done so in the past, he had relapsed on substances, and ultimately returned to his father. He said that intellectually, he understood the group's perspective, but on a visceral level, it was too scary to contemplate seriously alienating his father and being cast out on his own. The group leader appreciated the fact that Sean seemed to be calculating a cost/benefit ratio and was trying to decide if enduring his father's ongoing abuse was worth it. Was Sean's daily suffering part of the metric he was using in his calculation? What about the stalled career? The group leader wondered aloud what was preventing Sean from passing the nursing boards. After all, hadn't he passed multiple exams during nursing school? What might be getting in the way of his passing this one exam, which would give him entrée into a new career? Another group member chimed in, saying, "The way you respond so calmly and kindly to the rest of us in this group makes me feel like you would be an amazing nurse. Why don't you let yourself succeed?" Another member concurred, "I agree, with your warmth and personality, I think that you would be a great nurse. You have a very healing manner. And I know that if you stopped sabotaging your success, and actually practiced as a nurse, you wouldn't become a millionaire, but I suspect that you would be a lot happier than you are now." As the group session was coming to a close, the group leader asked Sean if he could look around the room and see the concern and compassion in the other men's eyes. Sean said that he could, and that he appreciated their kindness. The group leader suggested that because this was such a major issue for Sean, he hoped that he would continue to work on it with his individual therapist, and that he would also seek the support of his 12-step program to help deal with his fear of relapse as he learned to live independently.

Increased Ability to Titrate and Regulate Emotions

Survivors often avoid approaching their trauma memories for fear of the intense feelings these memories evoke. A group focused on understanding the impact of trauma can often elicit strong affective reactions, even with assurances that the details of traumatic memory will not be explored. Learning to tolerate the affect that this group elicits can be crucial in enabling survivors to tolerate affect when explicitly working through trauma memories in a later stage of recovery.

The present-focused nature of the TIG, in which group members do not talk about specific trauma memories, offers an opportunity to express and integrate some trauma-related affect in a more titrated and less overwhelming fashion. Practicing affect regulation begins with the check-in and grounding exercises at the beginning of each group and is repeated during the closing round. These exercises remind group members to pay attention to themselves and their bodies and encourage them to transition consciously and mindfully into and out of each group.

During the course of the group, leaders must actively, though compassionately, intervene to redirect group members who are beginning to share trauma memories in excessive detail. If detailed disclosure occurs, group leaders should normalize the desire to share more, but gently remind group members about the group guidelines and the purpose they serve. Group leaders may also suggest that individual therapy is a helpful place to begin processing specific memories that may be evoked.

Interventions aimed at helping group members stay present throughout the group are also essential in increasing the members' ability to regulate trauma-related affect. Group leaders should remain attentive to signs that members may be dissociating and intervene to help them orient back to the present moment. When the intensity of group content or affect increases to the point that multiple members appear overwhelmed or dissociated, it can also be helpful for group leaders to initiate a midsession check-in, in which group members say briefly how they are feeling and can get assistance from group leaders or other group members in recentering themselves.

As an example, as a group is progressing, Mary starts sharing about how angry she is at a culture that supports perpetrators. Her voice may be getting louder, and others are engaging as well, speaking angrily about how no one seems to care about victims. The group leaders notice, however, that Karen is seeming to withdraw. They may pause the discussion and note that it is really good to allow oneself to feel anger, but that they also want to stop and share an observation that maybe some members feel safe in expressing anger and maybe others feel less comfortable. This can lead to a dialogue about intensity and affect, and also about the fact that different individuals have different levels of tolerance for various emotions.

In another example of modeling tolerable affect and effective self-disclosure, in a recent group, a member said, "I was a really bad drug addict for a really long time. I abused cocaine, heroin, you name it, I tried it. I really loved that high feeling and just everything that went into getting ready to use." The group leaders felt concerned that evocative descriptions might be stirring up other members' memories or making substance use sound appealing. One of the leaders intervened by saying, "I think what Lisbeth is speaking about is that many survivors can identify with using something to self-medicate, whether it's food or television, or something else. Would people like to share about that?" The goal for the leaders would be to try to both contain, support, and empathize with the client, while at the same time asking the client to move on from giving excessive details. The hope is that this intervention would help the group member not feel exposed and vulnerable by sharing too much and also create a sense of commonality about how people have managed trauma-related emotions.

Enhanced Coping Skills

The relaxation or grounding exercises taught in the group, including practices such as diaphragmatic breathing, abbreviated progressive muscle relaxation, or simple yoga poses, can be used outside of the group as well. In addition, examples of healthy coping skills often come up throughout each session, as group members share strategies they have found helpful in their own recovery process. Often, group members report trying out skills that other members have suggested. Sometimes they may be more open to these suggestions than they may have been when a therapist suggested something similar. Hearing from another group member that a particular skill or strategy was helpful often comes across as more credible. In addition, it can serve as a reminder to try a coping skill when a difficult situation arises. Group members often "borrow" coping strategies from one another as a way of feeling connected. As group members internalize the group relationships, they report thoughts like "I remembered that X said when this happens to her, she does Y, so I tried it, and it helped."

Here is an example from a session on Self-Image/Body Image. The group is discussing the problem of intrusive symptoms that occur during consensual sex.

GROUP MEMBER 1: I don't want to be touched by anyone. The abuse will pop into my head.

GROUP LEADER 1: Have other people suffered from intrusions like that? (*Group members murmur yes.*) You don't want to be touched by anyone right now, so you just make it off limits. People have to figure out how to be in a sexual world in a way that works for them. Some people may take a moratorium from sex. Others may set really clear boundaries on what's okay. What's important is that consent means you can say yes or no to anything. That's really hard for any human being, but it's especially hard when your boundaries have been crossed. People have the right to say I want to stop.

GROUP MEMBER 1: What if you don't want to stop, but you just want to stop the intrusion?

GROUP LEADER 2: You could try stopping and talking about the intrusion to see if it's helpful—sometimes it might be, other times it may not be. You can stop and share that you don't want to stop but it's hard right now. When you're sleeping with someone you care about and who cares about you, it can often be helpful to have discussed these things in another time in another place with your clothes on.

GROUP MEMBER 3: Sometimes when I have something like that I want to stop for a minute. Sometimes I talk about the image I got, but a lot of times I just say, let's cuddle and talk about something different until I feel better.

GROUP LEADER 2: There are a lot of different ways. I think the basic idea is not to feel like your only option is to suffer through it and wait for it to be over, but to feel like you have options that can make you feel a little better than that. Whether it's stopping for a minute, stopping altogether, changing something in the environment that makes you more comfortable, asking your partner for help so you can deal with it together, do whatever it is that makes you feel like you have choices.

Increased Capacity for Safe Relationships

Disruption in relational and attachment capacities is one of the hallmark effects of chronic interpersonal trauma. Interpersonal violence simultaneously evokes emotional distress, undermines the capacity to regulate this distress, and compromises openness to social support by engendering distrust of others and shattering assumptions about the safety of the world (Charuvastra & Cloitre, 2008). Many symptoms of PTSD, such as avoidance and feelings of alienation, are themselves interpersonal in nature (Pearlman & Courtois, 2005). These very symptoms hinder trauma survivors from accessing the social support that could buffer the effects of the trauma.

These problems are even more enduring for survivors who have experience prolonged abuse at the hands of primary attachment figures. Adult survivors of childhood abuse frequently experience sensitivity to rejection, fears of abandonment, and ambivalence regarding trust and intimacy (Briere & Jordan, 2009). A great deal of research documents the unstable and chaotic relationships and high rates of revictimization in the complex trauma population (Cloitre, Cohen, & Koenen, 2006).

Safe attachment has been identified as an important indicator and goal of recovery (Tummala-Narra, Liang, & Harvey, 2007). However, many survivors struggle to find safe and graduated venues to learn to do this—they often try to forge new friendships at work or try to meet people in substance recovery meetings, only to find themselves back in relationships that repeat victim–perpetrator dynamics (Cloitre et al., 2006). They will often say, "I know I need to take it slow and begin with people who will understand what it's like. But where can I find such a place?" The highly structured format for peer interaction in the TIG allows for individuals to form safe connections and attachments with one another based on mutual support and reciprocity. The many interventions aimed at increasing the sense of safety and containment in the group also allow for group members to explore new ways of relating to others.

The group does not require a high baseline of relational capacities from group members, yet it offers ongoing opportunities for relational connection that group members tend to use increasingly as the group progresses. Often members are initially motivated to relate more directly to others by a sense of empathy and compassion for other group members that they do not feel initially for themselves. They are also often surprised to see that they have relational capacities, insights, and experiences that are of help to others, and that they can move back and forth between both giving to and receiving from the group. This sense of connection frequently crystallizes more explicitly during the last group meeting, in which group members get feedback from group leaders and group members on the progress they have made during the group and on the ways in which their contributions were meaningful and helpful to others.

The relationship of the co-leaders also serves as a model for healthy relating, in which leaders can share power equally and support each other, while also supporting the group as a whole, providing an experience of caring and respectful authority figures collaborating to promote the safety and growth of all participants. In this way, the group experience is designed to provide an alternate "template" that can be used by members to identify and cultivate safe and mutually supportive relationships outside of the group.

Increased Sense of Mastery and Empowerment

Prolonged and repeated interpersonal trauma can result in a pervasive sense of powerlessness and helplessness. Survivors often describe having a limited sense of personal agency and a general sense of futility about their ability to have control over their environment, personal circumstances, and future prospects. Over time, this fuels an enduring depression that can be more tenacious than frank PTSD symptoms. Many survivors doubt that they will ever be able to recover.

The TIG offers for many a first step toward an experience of mastery: a sense of pride in tolerating and completing a trauma-focused group. The group in turn can lead to an improved sense of self-efficacy. The mastery experience that the group celebrates is a powerful antidote to the feelings of helplessness attendant to victimization. It has been our observation that survivors leave the group with greater skills and confidence to accomplish goals in other domains of their lives.

At its core, the TIG is based on a principle of empowerment. It brings survivors out of isolation and silence and into connection with one another. It gives members choice and over time a greater ability to control their levels of disclosure regarding their traumatic past. It structures interactions in a way that conveys the notion that everyone has an equal right to be heard. It gives group members opportunities to contribute to the healing of others. Through a social and political analysis of interpersonal violence, the group helps members gain a broader understanding of what has happened to them, thereby transforming deeply shameful personal secrets into a collective experience of injustice. The group interventions and readings are clear in their stance that the perpetrator is solely responsible for violence and actively and compassionately recognize the limits of a child's capacity to cope with such violence. It has been our experience that members leave the group feeling that they have taken charge of their recovery. Group leaders talk with members about acquiring a sense of mastery in the group in the following explicit ways, which are highlighted as they occur in the group.

- By seeing that you can risk sharing things you have never been able to let others know before, and sometimes even letting yourself know something for the first time.
- By seeing that you have good ideas for others about strategies that have helped you in your recovery.
- By hearing how others have used therapy and recognizing your own successes.
- By being able to tolerate being in the group and by being helpful to others.
- By getting positive regard from others.
- By seeing that your feedback and presence in the group matters to others.

One member recently said at the end of the group, "I get it a bit clearer now. I can't change what happened, but I can change what happens from here. It's my job to believe that I can do a good job when I start college classes this year. I'll try not to feel like I'm 10 paces behind everyone else who's 15 years younger than me."

OVERVIEW AND DESCRIPTION
OF THE TRAUMA INFORMATION GROUP

Group Composition

The TIG generally has 8–10 group members and is ideally co-led by two therapists. However, the group may be led by a single clinician as well. Because the group is designed for people in early recovery, there are relatively few exclusion criteria. Members must be living in a safe environment and must not be actively psychotic. Sobriety is not a requirement, but prospective group members must agree not to come to the group in an intoxicated state. Group members must also be able to make a commitment not to act on suicidal ideation during the course of the group and must have a firm safety plan in place. Some groups require members to be in concurrent individual psychotherapy, but this requirement can be somewhat flexible, depending on the member's general stability and other social supports. Finally, group members should have had some basic experience of talking about their experience of trauma and its impact, even if this has only happened in individual therapy.

The Intake Process

Our current typical intake process involves a brief initial telephone interview followed by an in-person interview if it seems as though there is a match between the client and the group. After the in-person interview, with the prospective member's permission, the group leaders talk with her treatment team. We discuss each component of the screening process in greater detail shortly. Depending on the setting, this process could be modified to fit the setting and patient population.

Telephone Prescreening

We recommend an initial phone prescreening with each potential group member to discuss her interest and to provide some basic information about the group and the criteria for membership. Prescreening can save time and resources if there is clearly a poor match. Although these phone meetings tend to be fairly brief, we recommend that several key issues be addressed.

1. The group leader confirms with the client her interest in participating in a trauma group, communicates the time and duration of the group, and asks how she was referred.
2. The group leader provides some basic information about the group. In particular, the leader explains that it focuses on discussing the impact of one's traumatic experiences, rather than on revealing these experiences in detail. It is important that the leaders explain this aspect of group at the outset so that the client does not feel "set up" or "shut up" in the group. The group leader may say something like this:

"I'm glad you're interested in the group. Let me tell you a little bit about it. This is a group for people who have experienced trauma and want to get support related to how those experiences continue to affect them. Each week we will discuss a different way trauma impacts you as a survivor. In this group, people don't talk a lot about the details of what happened to them, but rather we focus on how the experience is still affecting them in the present. For example, if the topic of the session is trust, you might say, 'Because I was sexually abused by my uncle and my dad, it's really difficult for me to trust.' We would not want you to say, 'When I was 6, X happened, when I was 8, Y happened, so of course how can I trust anyone?' We limit the sharing of details in order to keep the experience manageable for everyone in the room. Do you have any questions about that?"

3. If the prospective member continues to express interest, the leader then goes on to discuss the criteria for participation. If the therapist and the client agree that this group sounds like a potentially good fit, the therapist will invite the client in for an in-person screening. If the client clearly does not seem appropriate for the group, she could be referred to other resources in the community.

In-Person Interview

Interest in Group Therapy

The group leader asks the potential group member to describe her interest in the group and what she might hope to accomplish by participating. For example, many clients have said, "My wish is to feel less alone; I probably won't trust anyone anyway, but I want to give it a try." Others have said, "My goal is to understand how the trauma has affected me."

If a prospective group member is likely to be in a minority—for example, the only person of color in the group—it is important that he or she is aware of it before agreeing to join. The leader may say, "I want you to know ahead of time that you may be the only person of color in this group. In the past we've had people in a similar situation, and this has not hindered their ability to find the group helpful, but it's your choice. How do you feel about this?"

Individual Therapy

It is not required that members be in individual therapy to participate in the TIG, although it is helpful if this is the case. However, this requirement is impractical in many treatment settings. The group leader asks the prospective client for more treatment history, with several important areas in mind. If the client is currently in therapy, she is asked to describe that treatment: how long she has been in treatment, how frequently she meets with the therapist, and what issues are being addressed. If the client is not currently in treatment, she is asked about other people to whom she can turn for support. A well-established recovery fellowship may serve this function. We would likely not accept into a group someone who is neither in individual therapy nor feels that she has *any* social supports.

What is important to assess here is how connected the prospective group member feels to her therapist and/or to other supportive people in her life, as this can be indicative of her capacity to form attachments and ultimately to benefit from the group. We also often ask the client herself what capacity she has to benefit from the group. A potential group member might say, "I could talk for an hour if you let me." The leader may respond with, "I'm so glad you told me that, because feeling that you are talking nonstop is not going to be helpful for the group or for you. Is there a way I can work with you to limit that without making you feel as if I'm trying to silence you?"

Trauma History

The client is asked to share some basic information about her traumatic past. Information to gather here could include a history of childhood physical or sexual abuse, sexual trafficking, witnessing or being victimized by domestic violence, or adult assaults. Gathering this information is important for several reasons. Since many clients in early recovery may not know how to talk about their histories, the group leaders can obtain a sense of the client's manner of doing so during the interview. Information about a client's trauma history is also significant for the group leaders in thinking about the group composition.

Safe Environment

The client's current living circumstances should be physically and emotionally safe (i.e., not being abused by a partner or child, not caring for a perpetrating parent). Some questions to include are:

"Who do you live with? Do you consider that a safe relationship?"
"Do you worry about being physically or emotionally harmed by your partner?"

Substance Abuse

To participate in the group, clients with serious substance abuse issues or a primary substance abuse disorder must make a commitment to monitor their drinking or use of drugs during the course of the group, and all members must make a commitment to come to group meetings sober. The group leaders can explain that although the TIG is structured and self-contained, being in a trauma group can evoke strong feelings and may exacerbate preexisting issues. If a client already uses substances to cope or self-medicate, she may find that her use increases during the course of the group. Our general goal in this part of the interview is to assess how serious a problem substances are for clients, how effective and functional they are in other parts of their lives, and how much risk their substance use is posing to them. Typically, the therapist asks, "Do drugs or alcohol feel like efforts at coping?" For those clients who struggle intermittently with substance abuse, they would be asked how realistic it is for them to participate in the group. Given that the TIG is an early recovery group, we do not exclude members from participating if they use substances. For example, if a member functions in the world, goes to work, and meets her responsibilities but uses marijuana at night for sleep, we would be likely to accept her into the group. It is important for readers of this guide to use their clinical judgment around these issues. For example, one client said this about her substance abuse:

> "Although I have been working on getting sober for years, I have yet to collect an entire 12 months of sobriety in a row. Invariably, I will get close, and then my father will reach out to me, or one of my siblings will tell me that my mother is wanting to be in touch with me, and wham, I'll lose it. It is like I can't let myself be successful with this, or anything."

In this case, the group leader suggested the possibility of joining the group, with the additional support of increased attendance at Alcoholics Anonymous (AA) and more frequent contact with her AA sponsor. The client made a commitment to sobriety for the duration of the group and was successful.

Safety Assessment

Many trauma survivors experience suicidal thoughts or self-harming urges. To be eligible for participation in the TIG, prospective group members should be able to commit not to act on such impulses and to tell the group leaders if they feel their symptoms are worsening. As with substance abuse, therapists should warn that thoughts of self-injury may be exacerbated by participation in an evocative group. However, if a client's suicidal thinking is relatively chronic and a daily struggle for her, we would generally accept her into the group only if she was in concurrent individual therapy. Some sample questions include:

> "Do you struggle with thoughts about wanting to hurt or kill yourself?"
> "Have there been times when you have acted on these thoughts?"
> "Have you been psychiatrically hospitalized? What circumstances led up to that?"
> "How do you manage these feelings when they come up? What prevents you from acting on them?"

In answer to this last question, prospective group members should be able to identify some positive reasons for living.

In this interview, we do not conduct a formal mental status exam. Since the majority of our clients do have individual therapists, we rely on the referring therapist to do an exam, as well as to provide diagnostic information and a sense of the client's presentation style. If the client does not receive individual treatment, it would be important to obtain diagnostic and risk information during the in-person meeting. If a client has also been diagnosed with a serious mental illness such as bipolar disorder, it would be important to ascertain how well managed the symptoms feel to the client. We would want the client to obtain psychopharmacology treatment and would get information about her symptoms from her prescriber as well.

Life Circumstances and Social Supports

When discussing with clients the fact that being in a trauma group can be difficult and evocative, the group leader asks prospective members who they turn to when they need emotional support. The leader inquires about friends, professional supports like therapists, and community connections, such as a religious community or recovery fellowship. The client should have some coping mechanisms in place that she can rely on during times of emotional distress, although given that this is an early recovery group, these ways of coping may be new and tentative. Sample questions are

> "When you have a bad day, what is the worst things get for you? How do you get through it?"
> "When you're having a tough time, what are some ways you deal with stress?"

Since the group is emotionally stressful, it is also important that the client not plan a major life change—such as a divorce, a move, or major surgery—during the course of the group. Leaders can inquire, "Are you anticipating any major life changes in the next 6 months?" The leader also explains that major life changes may make it hard for the prospective member to make the necessary commitment to the group.

Commitment to Reliable Attendance and Group Rules

The attendance policy of the group is explained: It is expected that members will attend each group and that they will arrive on time. Clients are asked directly if this is an expectation that they think they can meet. If a client says she can, but knows in advance that she will miss one session, this would be considered acceptable, but the client would be asked to inform the group in advance. Clients are told how important their presence is to the other group members; should they miss a week without notice, the other group members will tend to worry about them. Many trauma survivors do not realize how much they matter to others, and therefore do not appreciate that when they are absent from a group, they are actually missed.

Contact with the Individual Therapist, If Applicable

At the end of the screening interview, if it seems both to the group leader and to the client that this group may be appropriate, the decision about joining should be discussed with the client's individual therapist (if she has one). The client should be asked to sign a consent form permitting the leaders to be in touch with her therapist. The group leaders explain to the client the importance of working collaboratively with the client's individual therapist, so that her work in the group can be integrated into her individual work.

The group leaders will confer about the information provided by the individual therapist if there is one, and then, in consultation with the group supervisor, decide if the group is a good fit for the client. They then contact the client by phone to inform her about her admission to the group.

If the decision is made that the client is not ready for the group, the group leader will attempt to communicate the reason. In one clinical example, an individual therapist shared that the client had attempted many groups over the years, but had a history of missing many group meetings because of relapses with substance abuse. The group leaders shared their recommendation that the client focus on her sobriety and perhaps look into a substance-recovery intensive outpatient program and that she could consider the TIG at a later time once her sobriety felt more secure.

When a client is "screened out" of the group, as in the preceding example, the group leader should attempt to frame it in the context of the stages of trauma recovery. For a client to focus more intensively on her substance abuse recovery, for example, is another form of Stage 1 trauma work, which is about safety, stabilization, symptom management, and self-care. This is an important concept to communicate to the client, as shown in the following example.

In a recent group screening meeting, a potential group member shared that she had some ongoing legal struggles and had become sober in the past 2 months. The group leaders did not feel that this was the right time for her to pursue the group and shared their feedback with her in the following way:

> "More often than not, being in this group makes people more stirred up. We are guessing that the issues you have to deal with in court would already be contributing to that. Also, as you shared, you are newly sober. We don't want to risk your returning to a maladaptive coping mechanism because the group has 'stirred the pot.' Can you see it as part of your recovery process to wait and join the group when things are feeling more stable? In trauma recovery, it is so important to learn to pace yourself and see that as part of your recovery process."

There are also frequently situations in which clients are "screened out" because their histories are in some ways essentially different from the histories of the rest of the group members. For example, when group leaders meet with survivors of natural disasters or vehicular crashes, they communicate to them that this group may not be the right one for them, not because they are less traumatized, but because this particular group model focuses largely on the long-term impact of interpersonal violence, abandonment, and abuse. Similarly, we rarely "screen in" a homicide survivor because the dynamics of traumatic bereavement are unique and are not addressed sufficiently in this group model (see Aldrich & Kallivayalil, 2013, for a discussion of traumatic bereavement).

GENERAL FORMAT

The group meets for 10 weekly 60-minute sessions, thus requiring only a moderate time commitment both on the whole and for each individual session. One hour is generally considered to be a short time for a therapy group; this model, however, encourages a shorter group session. The primary rationale for this time frame is that we are attempting to offer a containing rather than an exploratory group, and this basic structure allows group members an opportunity for a titrated experience of tolerating affect related to their trauma history. At the same time, we have found it is long enough for group members to establish basic trust and connection with one another.

The group is structured so that meetings are predictable and so that interpersonal interaction occurs around content areas, not around details of traumatic experiences. The time limitation encourages the leaders and the members to attend strictly to the structure of the group and reflects the benefit of containment.

STRUCTURE OF GROUP SESSIONS

Each session is structured in a similar fashion, which helps make the group feel more predictable for group members. First, there is a brief check-in, followed by a relaxation/grounding exercise. Next, there is a topic-oriented discussion anchored by a psychoeducational worksheet. Finally, there is a brief closing round that emphasizes safety, allowing for a final reflection about the session and bringing closure to that week's group. Detailed descriptions of each group session are addressed in Chapter 3.

Check-In

The group begins with a brief check-in from each group member about how she is doing or feels about being in the group session that day. It allows each member to have an opportunity to bring her voice into the room immediately and, over time, to increase her comfort in participating. Many members report they have never been in a group context before and find the experience to be frightening. Some members find it difficult to participate in the large-group discussion, participating mostly in the "go-rounds." It may take them a number of weeks to find their voice in the group. The check-in guarantees that the co-leaders and the members have a clear opportunity to hear from one another. It also gently encourages those members who find it difficult to share to break their own self-imposed silence.

Relaxation

Next, one of the group leaders facilitates a brief relaxation exercise, aimed at helping group members to transition into the group and to be focused in the present moment. Grounding at the start of group can be particularly helpful for the many trauma survivors who struggle with significant hyperarousal, dissociation, or hypervigilance. Members who find the exercises helpful can use them outside of the group as well.

While many people find the relaxation exercises enjoyable, survivors who need to maintain some degree of vigilance in order to feel safe may have trouble with them. Having the option to participate with their eyes open may make the exercises more tolerable for some group members. Others may opt to just sit quietly during this time.

There are two types of relaxation exercises that are generally offered. The first is a form of progressive muscle relaxation combined with breathing. Members are usually asked to close their eyes, but are always given the option of keeping their eyes open. During this exercise, the leaders speak in a gentle, calm voice and exaggerate the sound of their breath. They then guide group members through tensing and relaxing different parts of their bodies. The second type of relaxation exercise involves gross motor movements. During this exercise, members may have their eyes open or closed. Leaders guide members through stretching and rotating different parts of their bodies. The purpose of this second exercise is to help members feel increasingly present in their bodies and to feel that their bodies are working for them. A cognitive component is included in both exercises, in which each member is encouraged to recognize the continuing work on their recovery that they are doing by coming to the group.

Topic/Worksheet Discussion

After this introductory phase, the group focuses on that session's topic-oriented discussion. The topics selected were chosen because they address important areas relevant to traumatic impact and recovery in both the research literature and in the clinical experience accumulated in the VOV Program. In each session a worksheet is used in conjunction with the topic. Group members are given the worksheet so that they can follow along as the co-leaders read. Group leaders take turns reading short sections of the worksheet and together facilitate discussion among group members after each piece of text is read. Group leaders take responsibility for reading to avoid situations in which group members may experience performance anxiety when reading or suffer anxiety because they have poor literacy skills or speak English as a second language. We have also had group members who have developmental and cognitive disabilities and, in these cases, we have shared the worksheets with their individual therapists so that they can integrate the information into their work and members can come to the group meetings prepared.

The group begins by exploring the broad impact of trauma and posttraumatic stress on various dimensions of experience, such as cognitive, spiritual, and emotional experience, and other trauma-related symptomatology. This topic is addressed first because it provides an organizing framework and offers an introduction to many different concepts about trauma and recovery in the most general and inclusive way, instilling a sense of affiliation and cohesion for group members. The topics then address safety and self-care in Session 2, and trust in Session 3. Once a greater degree of group cohesion—as measured in members' greater participation and ability to relate to one other—has been established, the more difficult and evocative topics of shame and self-blame, anger, and body image are approached. The final sessions (relationships and connections to others and making meaning of the past) help by offering a framework for continued recovery and growth.

Generally, each worksheet begins with a section describing what a child in a family with healthy boundaries would experience in the course of development. If the subject under discussion is body image, we would discuss how a baby learns to recognize that others will attend to his or her need for comfort, warmth, and nurturing. The worksheet then covers how children need encouragement about their physical activity and abilities and the affect that it has on developing a healthier body image.

Following this discussion of healthy development, the worksheet addresses the impact of trauma. For example, staying with the topic of body image, the worksheet describes how abused children may have been given overt shaming messages about their bodies being ugly or dirty. Or they may have learned to understand that something is wrong with their bodies because of the pain (or even pleasure) they experienced as a result of the abuse. The worksheet then describes the experiences of adult survivors. Cultural and political messages regarding body image are also addressed. For example, many survivors say, "My body always feels wrong because of the abuse I experienced." The leaders may respond by asking the group members if they think women who are not survivors of abuse are immune to this feeling. This question may lead to a discussion of the exploitative cultural messages that affect all women and may help to normalize some of the problems that survivors face.

As leaders read the worksheet, they stop periodically for discussion, elaboration, or clarification. Session-by-session guidance on how to do this is detailed in Chapter 3. During this segment of the group, some members may participate more than others. There is generally less hesitancy to join in as the group progresses. The worksheet ends with a number of related questions for the members to consider. Members can take their worksheets home to review and can bring them to individual therapy if they so choose, but there is no "homework" requirement.

Group members find commonality in sharing their posttraumatic symptoms and relational difficulties. The group is often described as a laboratory where people are encouraged to bring their problems and take some controlled risks in sharing. When they have been able to share successfully with others in the group, they can try to do this in their lives outside as well.

The "Go-Round" versus Open Discussion

Over the course of the group, discussion and reaction to the worksheets become more spontaneous as group members become more comfortable with one another. Leaders employ two main strategies to invite equitable participation and to ensure that everyone has a voice in the room. One is called the "go-round": After reading a paragraph from a worksheet, a leader might say, "Okay, why don't we go around the room. Can everyone say a little about her reaction to this paragraph about self-blame? Let's start with Member 1."

The "open discussion" is different in that it less explicitly asks everyone to contribute; rather, it encourages people to "jump in" as they wish to respond to a question and allows them also to respond to each other's questions. The leader might ask, "What do people think about what we just read about body image? Can anyone relate to it?"

The benefits and challenges of each type of intervention are obvious; in the "go-round," every member's voice is brought into the room, but it can at times feel prescriptive and clunky; the open discussion is more freewheeling and natural, but it runs the risk of having some members dominate the discussion and can lead to more conflict between members.

Closing Check-In

When the discussion of the worksheet is completed, or when only a few minutes are left until ending time, the group leaders call for a brief closing round, in which group members each say how they are feeling at the end of group, whether they feel able to maintain safety and self-care throughout the coming week, and whether they will be back for the next meeting. The check-in allows group members to reflect on their experience, provides group leaders important information about risk, and encourages a continued commitment to the group.

Given that there may not have been a great deal of detailed sharing in the room (especially in the early sessions), the closing check-in conveys an expectation to disclose a lack of safety so that group leaders can intervene. This action assures all members that their safety is of primary concern and will be monitored, as these groups accept many members who constantly struggle with addiction, self-harm, and suicidal thoughts. It also allows each member to leave knowing that her fellow group members will be attended to.

Members who are unable to guarantee that they are safe are asked to stay with the leaders, who will assess the situation and take whatever action might be needed to establish a safety plan. Often a call to a supportive person, friend, AA sponsor, or therapist will be sufficient. The fact that the group leaders noticed and took the time to intervene can often be quite meaningful for survivors who are accustomed to hiding their distress and bearing it in isolation.

CONCLUSION

In this chapter, we have reviewed the structure and format of the TIG and drawn connections between this structure and the goals of the group. These goals include providing an increased understanding of the impact of trauma, decreasing isolation and shame, and increasing group members' capacity for self-compassion, emotional regulation, and coping. The clinical examples provided in this chapter are meant to offer "experience-near" illustrations of how creating a safe and predictable structure in the group, providing psychoeducation, and encouraging progressive self-disclosure can increase a sense of connection among group members. We have also discussed some clinical guidelines for both phone and in-person screening that can be modified or adapted based on the setting and the population. In the next two chapters, we outline the nuts and bolts of running the TIG, with session-by-session instructions and illustrations.

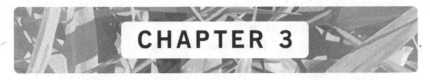

CHAPTER 3

Structure and Content of Sessions 1 and 2

This chapter provides an overview of the session-by-session content of the TIG and a guide for the development of the interpersonal process. In each of the sessions, we present the topical worksheet, concrete ideas about how to elicit and deepen discussion, common themes for the group leaders to highlight from the day's topic, and interventions that can help build group trust and cohesion. We recommend following the session-by-session outlines, particularly for newer clinicians or those unfamiliar with the content of the worksheets. Bear in mind that these outlines are not intended to be prescriptive or read word-for-word, and we expect that the co-leaders' natural therapeutic style will influence the wording and the delivery. This chapter presents the material for Sessions 1 and 2.

SESSION 1: THE IMPACT OF TRAUMA: POSTTRAUMATIC STRESS REACTIONS

The first session of the TIG accomplishes a number of tasks, including welcoming and introducing the group members, reviewing both the rationale and the structure of the group, explaining the ground rules, introducing the day's topic, and beginning to establish a sense of safety and trust among group members. Group leaders typically invite members into the group room at the same time. It is important that the room be prearranged with chairs in a circle for each member and co-leader, that lighting and temperature concerns be addressed, and that care is taken to minimize outside noise or disruption. Co-leaders should also take care of any disability accommodations requested by individual members. The leaders typically sit across from each other to maximize the visual perspective of the members and facilitate communication between them.

The topic for the first session, "The Impact of Trauma," educates the group members about the myriad ways their current functioning may be impacted by their traumatic experiences. Because all group members are suffering from trauma-related symptoms, this topic begins to establish a sense of commonality among them. We have found that the first worksheet outlining symptoms and reactions reduces group members' anxiety by allowing them to focus on something tangible and by providing a point of reference for discussion.

Session Outline

1. Introduce leaders and group members.
2. Review the schedules.
3. Inform group members about group structure and sharing.
4. Explain the guidelines.
5. Distribute paperwork.
6. Do a second round of introductions.
7. Present and discuss the topic.
8. Conclude with a closing check-in.

Content of the Session

The content of the session is described in detail below. We have included the main points the group therapists should attempt to cover in simple and direct language that is similar to how we have historically conveyed the material in the group. We expect the therapist will pause and ask if there are questions as she goes along, and we offer specific guidance about how to generate discussion.

1. Introduce Leaders and Group Members

After introducing themselves, the therapists will ask the members to state their first names and say a few words about themselves, such as where they live, who they live with, and how they spend their time during the day. Leaders should emphasize that this introduction should be about three to four sentences. The purpose of this opening check-in is to have everyone's voice be present in the room. The therapists clarify that this is only a brief introduction, and that more will be shared over time. Leaders may say:

> "At this time, we would like to give you a chance to introduce yourselves to one another. It is really up to you what you would want to share—just take a minute or two. You might say something about where you live, what you do with your time, whether you've been in group treatment before. Three or four sentences would be fine."

A typical introduction by a member might be "Hi, my name is Lisa. I live in Cambridge, I'm 45, and I work part time in a school. I came because my therapist thought this group would help me. I am very nervous. This is my first group."

Leaders can contain excessive talking by saying something like, "There will be lots of time to share more about yourself. This check-in is just to make you a little more known in the room right now." The co-leaders also introduce themselves and acknowledge the group members' accomplishment in taking the important step of coming to the group.

2. *Review of Day's Schedule and the Schedule of Sessions*

The group leaders outline the schedule for the first session as follows:

> "Now that we've introduced ourselves, I'd like to explain what will happen in the rest of this session. First, we are going to review the schedule of sessions and talk about the structure of the group. Then, we are going to explain the type of sharing involved in this group and outline some guidelines for group participation. We will then allow time for any questions or concerns you might have. Next, we will go through the first topic, 'The Impact of Trauma.' [Other group leader] and I will take turns reading the topic and we will take time to talk about it. We will end with a closing check-in."

The group leaders will also read through the schedule of sessions, pointing out any weeks missed because of vacations, holidays, and so on. This gives the group a sense of predictability and advance planning that can be calming and containing.

3. *Explain the Structure of the Group*

> "In this group we will be talking about the different ways in which your traumatic experiences have affected and still are affecting your lives. This group is unlike some other groups you may have been in, as it provides a lot of concrete information that we then discuss together. We will meet for 1 hour each week, except for holidays, as indicated on the schedule. Each session we will begin with a brief opening check-in to see how people are doing. We will then do a short relaxation exercise. The purpose of the exercise is just to help us transition from our day and focus on being in the room together.
>
> Because we have so much to cover in the first session, we will not do the relaxation exercise today and will talk more about it next week. After the relaxation exercise, we will introduce the day's topic. As you can see from the schedule, each week we will have a topic that we will discuss. The topics are presented in an organized way, with more difficult topics presented toward the end of the group when people feel more comfortable with one another. [Other group leader] and I will take turns reading the worksheet, stopping at times to see people's reactions and responses. At the end of the group, we will have a closing check-in to see how people are doing. The purpose of the closing check-in is to allow us to know that everyone is safe before leaving the group. If at some point in the group you don't feel safe, please let us know.

"Before we get into the ground rules, I would like to say a bit about the type of sharing that we encourage in this group. The goal of this group is to provide you all with a better intellectual and emotional understanding of how the traumatic events you have been through have affected your lives. So that everyone can benefit from the group, we need to establish a safe environment. Often, for people who have been traumatized, hearing the explicit details of someone else's traumatic experiences can be overwhelming and upsetting. For this reason, we ask that people talk about how their traumatic experiences are affecting them *today* rather than going into detail about their past experiences."

In this section, we are trying to model a very complicated challenge: how members can be real and authentic in the group without overwhelming themselves or others. In our experience of running this group, we have begun to realize that this is always a challenging part of the group experience. Group leaders cannot ultimately know or control when group members may have intense emotional reactions. For example, in a recent group, group members were deeply distressed by a member sharing that he used to eat out of a dumpster, something neither the sharing member nor the leaders expected. Group leaders should pay attention to all the members and learn to "read" the room, knowing that distress and dissociation may be unavoidable in the group. Leaders should explain this in a matter-of-fact way and encourage members to let them know when they are distressed. Knowing that such reactions are commonplace helps members feel less pathologized.

The group leaders may continue:

"Often when we talk about the type of sharing encouraged in this group, people become anxious about saying something wrong or inappropriate. We know that it is difficult for many people to learn to share in the way we ask you to do here, and that for many of you it may not feel right at first. If you start saying something that sounds too specific, we'll jump in. We don't want you to feel criticized; we are working on being here safely together."

The therapists should ask for questions at this point. Some members may be very anxious about the possibility that they may say the wrong thing during the group. If this concern is raised, the group leader should explain that all the group members will be learning how to talk about their histories, finding a balance between too little and too much sharing. If a member does begin to go into her trauma history in too much detail, the group leaders will stop her and ask her if she can summarize what she needs to say: "Denise, I'm going to stop you here. I know this is really painful, but I want to make sure that you talk about this in a way that's not overexposing for you and is bearable for other people in the room."

4. *Explain the Guidelines*

The therapists should then go on to explain the guidelines of the group. Group guidelines include confidentiality; mutual respect; no out-of-group contact during the course of the group; how to step in and step out of group discussions; and ground rules with respect to safety, food and drink, and lateness and absences. It is often helpful to have these guidelines typed out on a sheet of paper that you can pass out to members. A sample handout is included in Appendix B.

Attendance

"Group members are encouraged to attend every group. If you are unable to attend a group, please let us know in advance so other members will not worry. You can leave a message for _____ at _____ or _____ at _____."

Food and Drinks

"There is no food allowed in the group. Drinks are okay. Food can be distraction and a sensitive issue for other group members."

Often, therapists will observe group members nodding to this last statement. If the leaders observe members responding to this, they may say:

"I can see some nods. Clearly there is a connection for many survivors between having a trauma history and having struggles with food. During the course of the group, we will get to address this in more detail. We hope that having no food in the room provides a sense of safety for those who struggle in this area."

Confidentiality

"We want you to talk about the group with your supports as much as you want to, but we want you to do it in a way that isn't identifying to anyone. We don't want to you say, 'Jane Smith had a really good idea about dealing with flashbacks.' We'd rather you said that there is a woman in the group who struggles with flashbacks from her abuse and she takes a lot of walks to help her feel better. I thought that was a great idea and decided to try it too."

In individual therapy, the word *confidentiality* may have been used but in a different way—usually to refer to the responsibility of the therapist. In addressing this issue here, the group leaders are illustrating how to create a confidential and safe space along with a feeling of group affiliation.

No Planned Out-of-Group Contact

"Were you to run into each other outside the group, we ask you to maintain each other's privacy and not identify how you know each other. Planned outside contact between group members while the group is going on is not permitted. The reason for this is that it can create complicated dynamics that make it difficult for the group to work well."

Safety

"In order to participate in the group, individuals need to be in safe living situations, to be able to maintain sobriety, and not to be self-harming. If you are struggling with these issues, we will check with you (and your therapist if you have one) to evaluate the advisability of remaining in the group."

Step In, Step Out

"There are going to be times when we go around the room and ask each person to comment about a given topic, and there will be other times where we open up the floor for a more spontaneous larger discussion. In these situations, we ask that you monitor your talking and 'step in and step out'—so you can both contribute and give space to others."

5. Distribute Paperwork

The group leaders will pass out information packets that include their names and phone numbers, a schedule of the 10 topics, and the group guidelines.

6. Do a Second Round of Introductions

Because group members are often so anxious at the beginning of the group, we have them introduce themselves in more detail at this point—after they have been given more information about the structure of the group.

> CO-LEADER 1: So now we will transition to our opening check-in. As you all know, I am Sam and it's very good to see you all here. I imagine that there are many feelings in the room; starting a group of this kind is very anxiety producing for most people.
>
> CO-LEADER 2: Yes, so we want to congratulate you all for taking this step to be here and appreciate that there may have been many challenges in getting here today. I am Sophie.
>
> CO-LEADER 1: We will have a very full group tonight. Sophie will outline how we typically begin each group, which is with a check-in or opening round.
>
> CO-LEADER 2: The check-in is a brief opportunity, just a minute or so, for each of you to say a sentence or two about how you are feeling as you start each group session. It is meant to help you to transition into the group and to bring your voice into the room. For example, you may want to share what kind of day or week you are having or where you are emotionally as you begin the group today. It is very important that every group member participate in this opening round in some way. So, let's start with our check-in. Who would like to start?
>
> MARIA: I guess I'll go. My name is Maria. I feel like I'm jumping out of my skin a little. I can't believe I made it, but I'm here.

CO-LEADER 1: We're really glad you're here.

ANGELA: My name is Angela. Not sure what to say. I'm surprised to see so many people. I guess we all need the help!

CO-LEADER 2: Glad to have you here, Angela.

The opening round continues in this way until everyone has been reintroduced.

7. *Present and Discuss the Topic*

The therapists should distribute the first worksheet, "The Impact of Trauma: Posttraumatic Stress Reactions," explaining that they will take turns reading and will stop occasionally for discussion. It can be helpful to start with a discussion of "What is a traumatic event?" Members will often say, "To me it means horror" or "Trauma is something that should never happen to anyone anywhere." This discussion often leads to a common understanding and an early sense of cohesiveness in the group. Leaders should not expect to go through every symptom on this worksheet. Rather, leaders may choose certain sections and highlight them, for example, "How Trauma Affects How One Relates to Others."

The therapist could say, "This first worksheet is about the impact of trauma. For some of you, this may be a review and for others part of it may feel like new information. In my experience, almost everyone learns something new in reviewing this worksheet." The therapist will then begin reading the worksheet, while pausing to intersperse open-ended questions and clarifying comments.

Members are often unsure about how to label their experiences. They may say things like, "People tell me that what happened to me was abuse, but I think getting hit by your parents was just how you were brought up." Group leaders can respond by saying, "Having and developing a language that makes sense to you to describe your experience is really important. We are interested in how *you* feel about what happened to you."

If a group member does not like to use the word *incest*, or would rather say "sexual assault" instead of "rape," the leaders and the group members do not relabel their experiences for them. In keeping with our empowerment stance, we believe that trauma survivors need to develop their own language to describe their experiences.

As people continue to heal, they become more comfortable naming experiences and holding perpetrators accountable.

To work through the sections on common reactions, the leaders can focus on a particular topic and ask the members to mark with a pencil what reactions they can identify with. They should read slowly, looking around for reactions members share in common. The group leaders can also say, "In looking at the cognitive impact section of the worksheet, there are 11 items listed. How many of you checked more than 8?" At this point, the leaders can recognize the universality of the reactions and by expanding the question to "Which are the most relevant to you?" In response to a particularly relevant symptom, leaders may pause and say, "Look around the room. Every hand is up. Take a moment and look at each other."

Weeks later, when people are saying good-bye at the end of the group, it is not unusual for them to refer to this early and powerful experience of commonality. They often say that though they felt too overwhelmed to speak to it at the time, it rendered powerfully the shared experience of traumatic exposure.

At this point, it is helpful to do a "go-round" to get everyone's voice in the room. The leaders may say, "We're going to do a 'go-round' now. Pick one of the items that you feel you can really relate to and say something about it." Members in recent groups said in regard to their symptoms of hypervigilance, "Sometimes the slightest noise throws me into fight-or-flight, and I have to remind myself, I'm here, there's no danger" and "I get mad at myself for my jumpiness, even though I'm used to it, because it scares other people and it's embarrassing." As members go around, it is important to continue to highlight commonality.

Clarifying comments are designed both to spark discussion and deepen understanding of the topic. For example, a leader might say, "Many people have lots of symptoms and haven't really thought about how they relate to their histories. Can anyone explain how dissociation is connected to trauma?"

The following table outlines some specific themes that arise in relation to the first topic and offered some suggestions with regard to how group leaders may address them.

Themes	Clarifying Comments/Questions
Delayed versus immediate reactions to trauma Some people may experience these symptoms immediately after a trauma, while for others they may take years to appear.	The group leader may ask, "Can you share something about when your trauma symptoms began or when you realized that your symptoms had something to do with trauma?" At this point, members may say how "crazy making" it can be when all of a sudden these symptoms take over their lives. This can be a common bonding experience in the group. A member in a recent group said, "I thought I cut myself because I was crazy. The idea that people cut themselves because they are trying to deal with pain never occurred to me." Another member said, "I wish I had known 20 years ago that this was trauma when all these things started popping up. I thought there was something really wrong with me."
Why address the impact of trauma in clients' lives now?	Leaders may ask, "Has anyone ever thought that there might be some reason that they are more able to deal with their traumatic experiences now, compared with 5 or 10 years ago? "Sometimes it's adaptive not to address your history directly right away. For example, if someone was able to go to college and successfully get a job at a geographic distance from her family, it might be safer to look at this now, from a greater distance."
List of common reactions	"Is there anything on this list that is new to you? Something you hadn't thought about as being related to your trauma history?" A member recently said, "The idea that a 9-year-old could cut herself—I never thought it was trauma, thought I was just crazy. I didn't

Themes	Clarifying Comments/Questions
	tell anyone, I just thought I was nuts, and they would think I was nuts." Another member said, "I have these thoughts, these images, they pop up, and they're out of control. I don't know what the triggers are, there are so many."
The client asks, "How does X [e.g., difficulty making decisions] relate to my trauma history?"	Often other group members can be relied on to help explain connections between current symptoms and trauma history. Leaders might ask, "Does anyone have ideas about how X may relate to a trauma history?"

During this session, the group members will often mention different symptoms that they have that they hadn't realized were trauma related. Frequently group members will begin checking off symptoms they experience and comparing their reactions to other group members. This is often a point of real connection building in the group, as members discover that other people share their suffering. In recent iterations of the group, one participant said that while the other group members said they feared everything, she feared nothing. Reading through the list together made her realize that both reactions came from the same place. She said, "Fear is meant to keep you safe; if fear does nothing to protect you, the mechanism turns off." Another participant said in reference to how she used substances to keep the trauma memories at bay: "When I bottomed out from alcohol and finally got sober, I started walking straight into the trauma and saw how far back it went." I always wondered, "Why do I relate to these people's stories of abuse and horrible families I read about? I had told myself this never happened to me." The group leader responded, "People disconnect from what happened to protect themselves. Sometimes denial works, at least for a time, and sometimes it doesn't."

Isolation is a consequence of trauma that group members can often identify with. As one group member said, "My friends will ask if I'm still alive because I go and withdraw on them. I need people, but I push people away, but then I ask, why did they give up on me? But it makes sense; they leave after 6 months. They get tired of it."

Another participant agreed and said, "I'm a fake. . . . I was a class clown, life of the party. I wanted people to like me so much. I feel like I wear a mask the whole time, and if I'm not wearing a mask I don't want to be near people because what if they hate me without the mask." A group leader responded, "It can be hard to know how to let in the people who really matter to you. One of the reasons we offer this group is to provide a space for people to feel less alone, to say there are places to share and be safe." Another group member said, "I get that, but I feel more alone when I'm with people. I isolate to protect myself. People don't understand, they say, 'Just get over it!'"

At about 15 minutes before the end of group, the leaders should indicate how much time is left and bring the discussion to a close, emphasizing how people recover from trauma. They may say something like this:

"Recovery from trauma is a complicated process that takes time. There are many aspects to it—managing symptoms, learning to take better care of yourself physically, emotionally, and, for some, spiritually. Why don't we do another 'go-round'? This time, think about either one aspect of recovery that you feel you have achieved successfully or another in which you would like to make some progress."

In so doing, the leaders encourage the members to share self-care strategies and use the time to emphasize the importance of self-care in the recovery process. Doing so gets people's voices in the room, while encouraging them to see their successes with self-care and the possibility for change. Some examples of statements from group members at this stage are: "Food is my comfort, it's my drug, I gotta stop with the caffeine and the sugar, I need to work on eating well and I'm going to try to do that," or "I would love to set ambitious goals, but if I can just brush my teeth that would be great," or "The hard part is exercise; I don't like people seeing me move, it makes me feel really vulnerable." The leaders can gently help reframe some of these goals. For example, regarding the goal of eating better, a leader might say, "Would you like to try to focus on perhaps limiting sugar 1 day a week and see how that works for you?" It is important to end on a note of optimism. Leaders convey their knowledge that recovery is possible, their confidence that the group members are on the road to recovery, and their hope that members can feel some optimism for themselves.

Before starting the closing check-in, the leaders should make some summary comments about the first group. They might include saying something about how many of the group members seemed to share certain experiences or how, despite their anxiety, people were able to share how they were feeling. It is important to validate what an important step they have each taken in being part of the group.

8. *Conclude with a Closing Check-In*

The leaders should inform the members that they are interested in hearing briefly how each member is doing, whether she is safe leaving the group for the day, whether she plans to return next week, and how she is feeling as the session is ending. Members who are unable to guarantee safety are asked to stay briefly in the room. Sometimes a group member will ask, "What does safe mean? I don't know what safe is." The leaders can respond, "I'm glad that you asked. Safety can be a complicated word for trauma survivors. For our purposes today, we mean physical safety—that someone is not suicidal and not feeling that she wants to harm herself. We will talk more about safety next week."

At the end of the worksheet, there are additional questions and notes. Leaders may call attention to them before the members leave, saying, "There are some additional questions at the end of your worksheet. Feel free to read and think about them by yourself, or bring them to your individual therapy, or share them with someone who cares about you. There is no expectation of homework in this group, but the worksheets are yours to use during the week if you wish." Leaders may also want to warn members that this first group meeting may bring up memories and strong feelings during the course of the week and to reassure them that such reactions are normal and understandable.

SESSION 2: SAFETY AND SELF-CARE

The topic for the second group, "Safety and Self-Care," provides information to the group members about how difficulties in these areas may relate to their traumatic experiences. This topic is a natural next step for the discussion of trauma recovery that was begun in the first group session, since establishing safety and self-care are some of the important first steps in the recovery process. In this session, members are encouraged to identify ways they are or may feel unsafe or struggle to identify self-care strategies. They are also encouraged to share strategies for safety and self-care that have been helpful for them with other members of the group. As always, interventions in this meeting are intended to also build group cohesion and a sense of belonging for the group members.

Session Outline

1. Tie up loose ends from the first meeting.
2. Review today's schedule.
3. Introduce the opening check-in.
4. Explain and introduce the relaxation exercise.
5. Present and discuss the topic.
6. Conclude with a closing check-in.

Content of the Session

1. *Tie Up Loose Ends from the First Meeting*

Often, because of time constraints and scheduling conflicts, all the tasks for the first meeting do not get completed. Also, there may be new members who were not able to attend the first meeting. If this is the case, the group leaders will want to provide them an opportunity to introduce themselves and meet the other members at the start of the group.

2. *Review Today's Schedule*

If needed, at this time the leaders will offer information regarding possible member absences. After the roll call is complete, the group leader says:

> "I'm glad to see you here today. Before we go through the opening check-in and see how everyone is doing since last week's meeting, I would like to outline what we will be doing today. We are going to follow a schedule that will be the same each week from now on. First, we will start with a brief opening check-in like the one we practiced last time. Following that, we will go through a brief relaxation exercise. I will talk more about this after the check-in. Then we will distribute the handout on today's topic,

'Safety and Self-Care,' read through it together, and have a discussion on the topic. We will end with a closing check-in as we did last week."

3. *Introduce the Opening Check-In*

Since this is only the second week, we often have members introduce themselves again during the opening check-in. We ask members to say their names and say something briefly about how they have been feeling since last week or about how they feel about being back in the group. Often members will say something like "I was really anxious and didn't feel like coming this week, but glad that I'm here now." It is important for the group leaders to acknowledge again what a big step they have taken in returning to the group and normalize the fact that the first meeting may have stirred up trauma-related memories or feelings. At this stage in the group, it is particularly important to normalize group members' experiences by saying things like "Did other people find that a lot of difficult feelings came up? Maybe that they were not expecting?"

4. *Explain and Introduce the Relaxation Exercise*

Before introducing the exercise, leaders should clearly explain the rationale for it, as well as the fact that it is completely voluntary. Group leaders may say something like the following:

> "Now we are going to talk about the relaxation exercise. The purpose of this exercise is to help all of us separate from the stresses of the day and to orient to being present in the room together in as centered and focused a way as we can. Also, learning relaxation techniques has helped many people to deal with traumatic stress. That said, we are aware that many of you might not feel comfortable at first with the idea of participating in a relaxation exercise. Many of you may feel that you need to be hypervigilant—constantly on the alert for danger and aware of what is going on around you. We talked about this feeling in the first group meeting as one of the symptoms of posttraumatic stress. Hypervigilance is an understandable reaction to trauma and may in some ways have served you well. But hypervigilance is also associated with a level of anxiety that makes it difficult to sit still and be calm and curious in the present.
>
> "Though relaxing might feel scary, we want to create a safe space where people feel grounded, centered, and open to new ideas and feelings. At the same time, we want each of you to decide for yourself to what degree you are comfortable participating in these exercises. For example, you may want to participate in the exercise but may not feel comfortable closing your eyes. That's fine. Or you might decide just to sit quietly as we do the exercises. Learning to respect your individual comfort level is part of learning to keep yourself safe and taking care of yourself, fitting in with our topic today. Any questions?"

Group leaders should feel free to use relaxation exercises that are simple and with which they are comfortable.

5. *Present and Discuss the Topic*

The group leaders should hand out the worksheet, explaining that they will begin by reading the worksheet, stopping frequently for clarifying comments and discussion. For example:

> "In the last group, we first talked about the impact of posttraumatic stress and ended by talking about how people recover from trauma. If you remember, we discussed some strategies that help with the recovery process, such as addressing the need for sleep and getting regular exercise. This second worksheet is about safety and self-care. This is an important topic and a good way to start the second group because Safety and Self-Care are viewed as the foundations of the recovery process."

The therapists will then begin reading the worksheet, a couple of paragraphs at a time, while pausing to intersperse clarifying comments and questions to promote discussion and deepen members' understanding of the material. This session often involves members' reflections on how self-harm was a way to cope with pain. In recent groups, members said things such as "I never considered alcohol and drugs a danger. They saved my life. If I hadn't had them, I probably would have committed suicide by now," and "When I was very young, I knew I would be a drug addict before I even did drugs. I read an article about a kid who did drugs, and she said the pain she felt just went away when she did it and she could face herself and the day. I said to myself in that moment, that's what I need." The following table outlines some additional themes.

Themes	Clarifying Comments/Questions
How to define safety when you have never been or felt safe	"We just read how feelings of safety develop when children are responded to and cared for. How do people learn about safety when this is not the context they grow up in?" A member may say, "I don't know what safety is. I only know what not safe looks like." Another member recently said, "I intentionally put myself in unsafe situations because I felt petrified all the time anyway and I didn't know why. So you need the bad situation to kind of validate the feeling, if that makes sense."
Misperception of whose job it was to create safety—the caregivers' or the child's Group members often talk about how they blame themselves for not keeping themselves safe, *even when this was clearly impossible*, particularly when they were children. They might also talk about how they wanted to control	Leaders can facilitate members' understanding of why they gave up on safety—and how now that they are no longer in a traumatic situation, they have the opportunity to make themselves safe. Leaders might say, "It sounds like many of you gave up on safety in childhood because you had no choice given how abusive your families were. You might believe your safety is not important because you don't matter somehow. Does anyone of you feel like you've also given up on safety in adulthood?"

Themes	Clarifying Comments/Questions

and make the environment safe for others, such as younger siblings, when that was not possible. In some cases, group members may have made themselves the target of abuse in an attempt to make the environment safe for others—for example: "If I go along with my uncle's abuse, he won't abuse my younger sister." Often, these attempts to create safety did not achieve the desired goal. As a result, many trauma survivors may have given up on the idea of safety altogether.

Members might say that they feel there is no use trying to be safe when anything, particularly bad things, can happen at any time. Talking about beliefs about safety can then lead to a discussion of what can be done to keep safe and what cannot." A group leader might say, "Of course something might happen to us no matter how much we protect ourselves. Does that mean we can't protect ourselves at all?"

Identifying ways you may be unsafe or do not care for yourself

We have found that a discussion of this topic often brings up anger for the group members—usually directed at the parent or caregiver who was not frankly abusive but did not protect them. It is important to pause here for some discussion, and also to remind group members that anger will be addressed more directly in a later session.

"Why is self-care so challenging? How do people feel it is related to how you feel about yourself?" Here the group leaders can use examples from the worksheet and their own clinical experiences of how clients use unsafe coping mechanisms, such as cutting, substance use, or risky sexual encounters. They can also talk about changes these clients made to keep themselves safe.

Identifying destructive coping strategies, such as substance abuse and self-harm

Often members will bring up the fact that using certain coping strategies, such as drinking, which are at times harmful, make them feel better in the short run. This is a critical discussion to have so that group members can experience commonality with others, which can help dilute the sense of shame they often feel for using these strategies. The group leaders should explain how and why people who have been traumatized develop coping strategies that seem self-destructive. The group leaders must emphasize that the use of these strategies is understandable in the context of a traumatic history and that members use these strategies because they provide relief—*but* that these strategies have a cost. The key for survivors now is to find strategies that work and help them cope without the same cost.

Recently, as group members read the section on self-destructive coping mechanisms and substance use, the

Themes	Clarifying Comments/Questions
	group leader asked, "Who else has self-medicated? No one says 'I want to be an addict,' we use it to change an emotional state we are in." A group member responded, "All I wanted to do was behave normally and I needed drugs to do that. I wasn't trying to escape, I was trying to be normal. Another member agreed, "If you don't medicate, you feel totally out of control."
Identifying alternative safe coping strategies	This is often a point where members can be very helpful to each other. Leaders might ask, "Has anyone developed new ways of coping with overwhelming feelings that seem to work for her?" or "Mary has said she doesn't know what to do when she feels angry at herself. Does anyone have suggestions?"
Identifying self-care strategies	Group members often have difficulty identifying ways in which they can take care of themselves *now*. Group leaders may ask members to go around the room and say one thing they do for themselves that makes them feel good, such as attending an AA meeting, reconnecting with a friend, reading, cooking a healthy meal, or spending time with a pet. At the end of the group, leaders can ask members to state one self-care and self-affirming activity they will do for themselves over the next week.

6. *Conclude with a Closing Check-In*

As in Session 1, the therapists should inform the members that they are interested in hearing how each member is doing and whether she is safe leaving the group for the day. Members who are unable to guarantee safety are asked to stay after the session.

CONCLUSION

In this session-by-session guide for Sessions 1 and 2, we provide concrete illustrations of the basic tasks of the early stages of the TIG: welcoming and introducing the group members, reviewing both the rationale and the structure of the group, explaining the ground rules, discussing confidentiality, introducing the day's topic, and beginning to establish a sense of safety and trust among group members. We also provide a guide for beginning to develop a containing interpersonal process. The next chapter details the session-by-session content for Sessions 3 to 10, which follow a somewhat altered structure.

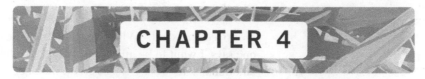

CHAPTER 4

Structure and Content of Sessions 3–10

Sessions 3–9 of the TIG follow an identical session outline; only the topic changes from week to week. Specific topic-related content for each session is also discussed.

GENERAL SESSION OUTLINE

1. Introduce the opening check-in.
2. Explain and introduce the relaxation exercise.
3. Present and discuss the topic.
4. Conclude with a closing check-in.

CONTENT OF THE SESSION

1. Introduce the Opening Check-In

We continue to do an opening check-in each week so that each group member has the opportunity to have her voice heard in the room. Depending on how well the sessions go from week to week, we may ask a question to initiate the opening check-in—for example: "We noticed last week's topic was particularly difficult for many of you. When you go around, maybe each of you could say briefly how you were doing last week after our session." Or we might ask members to talk about how it feels being back this week. Our purpose in doing this is to give members permission to talk about their positive and negative reactions to the group. Often an individual member may feel as though he or she is the only one who has a certain reaction to the group. During the opening check-in, this member will often find that many other members are experiencing similar feelings. The expression of these common feelings increases group cohesiveness.

2. *Explain and Introduce the Relaxation Exercise*

The relaxation exercise is introduced following the opening check-in as described on page 44 in Chapter 3. Group leaders will need to use their clinical judgment in varying the exercise according to group members' needs, abilities, or disabilities, so that all members benefit. Suggestions are available on pages 29–30.

3. *Present and Discuss the Topic*

As before, the group leaders hand out the worksheet for the week's topic, explaining that they will read the worksheet a paragraph at a time, stopping for clarifying comments and discussion. Specific issues relevant to each topic will be presented below.

4. *Conclude with a Closing Check-In*

As in Sessions 1 and 2, the therapists should inform the members that they are interested in hearing how each member is doing, whether she plans to return the following week, and that she is safe leaving the group for the day. Members who are unable to guarantee safety are asked to stay after the group session.

SPECIFIC TOPIC-RELATED CONTENT FOR SESSIONS 3–9

Session 3: Trust

Trust is a complicated issue for trauma survivors, and being in a group setting can provide an unparalleled relational opportunity to address their conflicts around trust. We can speculate that some evidence of members' developing trust will make itself known by their behavior in the group: whether they attend regularly and on time and appear to feel contained by the group process. Leaders help build this trust by caring for the group in a predictable way (e.g., being on time, providing a structure and containment, returning phone calls from members, and acknowledging absences).

Being traumatized violates an individual's basic sense of trust—in others, in the world around her, in God or a higher power, and in herself. Trust is therefore an issue for all trauma survivors to some degree. Individuals who have been traumatized in childhood may find that they never developed a sense of basic trust in the outside world. Those who have been exposed to prolonged and repeated trauma as adults may find that whatever trust they had in others has been shattered.

Trauma survivors often do not feel that they can even trust themselves. If others have not believed their stories, survivors may doubt their own memory. Furthermore, one of the most robust predictors of being victimized in adulthood is having been victimized in childhood. Survivors who have been victimized by multiple perpetrators may be left feeling that they can't trust their own judgment. The following table illustrates some additional themes.

Themes	Clarifying Comments/Questions
The definition of basic trust	Survivors who were traumatized outside their families and/or as adults may feel that at one time they knew what basic trust was. Survivors who suffered from familial abuse may never have known what basic trust is. Leaders should read the first two paragraphs of the handout and then explore with members what basic trust is. Leaders can then help members think about whether or not they developed basic trust in their families of origin. "Is basic trust something that is familiar to anyone? Or is it a totally foreign concept?"
Learning basic trust	Leaders can help members think about how they can learn basic trust. "How does someone learn basic trust if she didn't grow up in a family that taught or showed it?"
Common problems with trust Survivors commonly oscillate between extremes in terms of trust. On the one hand, they may trust no one. On the other hand, they may be too trusting. Also, survivors have been hurt so many times that they often do not trust themselves or their own judgment.	Leaders should encourage members to talk about the common problems with trust. In our experience, members will often initiate a discussion of these problems themselves. If they do not, leaders might want to say, "Many survivors oscillate between extremes when it comes to trust. They either trust too soon and get hurt or don't trust anyone. Sam, I see you nodding. Where do you find yourself when it comes to trust?" Members often share that they have a mark on their foreheads that says "sucker." A discussion about how others feel like this can be very affirming.
Recognizing ways in which survivors can rebuild trust	As just mentioned, members might say that they have learned never to trust anyone, so they don't. Leaders can help them recognize how they may trust selected others—a good friend, perhaps a therapist, or other group members. Any survivor who joins the group is showing some ability or willingness to trust. Trust is not an all-or-nothing proposition.
The impact of a betrayal of trust—relationships with others	"How do you think having your trust betrayed like that has affected your relationships with other people? Do any of you find you trust too much when you shouldn't, or not at all when you should give someone a chance? Do you push people away?"

Themes	Clarifying Comments/Questions
The impact of a betrayal of trust—not trusting yourself Trauma survivors may lose trust in themselves for many reasons. Because they have trusted people in the past who have hurt them, they may not trust their judgments about people. Because of the splintered nature of their memories, amnesia, and/or a tendency to dissociate, they may not trust their experience. Given their tendency to self-medicate with alcohol, drugs, or food, they might not trust themselves to take care of their own basic needs. Because their feelings are so out of control, survivors might not trust themselves to be safe.	"We've talked about how trauma has affected your ability to trust others—what about your ability to trust yourself? Sometimes when you are hurt by so many people you stop trusting your own judgment—has anyone felt that way?" Members will often discuss how their dissociative symptoms have affected their ability to trust themselves. They may say, "It's not even just the world, it's also yourself. You can't rely on your own memory, like you're black-out drunk but you're not. It feels unsafe because you can't trust yourself." Depending on how the discussion proceeds, leaders might say, "Sometimes people in this group say that they can't trust how they will act with other people because their feelings are so out of control. Does this sound familiar?"

Session 4: Remembering

The session on remembering is often a difficult one. This is in part because for most trauma survivors remembering is associated with overwhelming feelings and therefore often an increase in symptoms.

Readers who see clients individually can attest to the fact that "remembering" is a frequent theme in therapy. Many patients come to therapy with the express wish "to remember what happened to me" or say things like "I know what happened and that was bad enough, but I just know there was more. If only I could remember what that was, things might make more sense to me," or "If it was that bad, why can't I remember? I have no memories of my early childhood—nothing before age 9." Others may feel preoccupied with images and thoughts of the past, saying, "I spend so much time thinking about the past, I don't enjoy the present, it's just a blur."

Group leaders can create a calming atmosphere to contain the tension many group members feel about remembering by explaining that "remembering everything" is not the goal; rather, it is important over time to feel that one has a coherent life narrative. Leaders may say:

"Many trauma survivors have difficulty remembering the details of what happened to them. This is normal. It might have been adaptive not to remember. Perhaps not remembering lets you get on with other things—going to school, working, moving out of your family's home, having a family of your own. People remember in many different ways, at different times in life. It's okay not to remember everything. What's important now is trying to take in as much as we can about the present moment."

While keeping these issues in mind, the leader will then begin reading the worksheet, while interspersing clarifying comments and questions as illustrated in the following table.

Themes	Clarifying Comments/Questions
Feeling a lack of control over the remembering process One of the hallmarks of trauma is a lack of control over the remembering process. Survivors often feel at the mercy of memories about their experience that intrude both while they are awake and while they are asleep.	Group members often find it helpful to be reminded that intrusive memories in the form of nightmares or flashbacks are a common outcome of being traumatized, and that when they have these symptoms they are not "going crazy." A recent group member said, "Any memories I do have are so disconnected, I feel like it still happened to 'she' versus me. I can feel more compassion toward others because I don't question them; because I don't have access to these years it's hard to understand why I am this way. I don't necessarily want to feel better, I need to feel my experience. I just want to stop oscillating between it happened, it didn't happen." The group discussion can be framed so that members learn techniques for gaining some control over their memories. A group leader might say, "It sounds like many of you have felt out of control when it comes to remembering. Has anyone found something she can do that helps her feel more in control?" The leader may have to offer an example such as: "For example, in another group, a member said she stopped going to violent movies because they made her have flashbacks."
Overwhelming feelings and a great deal of distress brought up by remembering Remembering can bring up feelings of terror, hopelessness, shame, guilt, rage, and so forth—any emotion that might be associated with being victimized can be brought up in remembering. Learning to manage these feelings is an important part of gaining control over the remembering process.	Group members should be encouraged to think about when they have effectively managed these feelings and when they have not. Techniques for managing overwhelming feelings should be discussed. Some techniques members have suggested include practicing breathing and relaxation techniques (for anxiety), hitting a pillow (rage), challenging thinking patterns (hopelessness, guilt), and DBT self-soothing skills.
Clients say, "Should I remember everything? Is it bad that I don't remember everything?" This question often comes up in this session. Some group members may be on a quest to remember "everything." Often this quest	Leaders may wish to point out that no one remembers everything about their lives and open the question up for discussion in the group about the meaning behind this wish to remember more. "Do people feel they need to remember everything to get better? Why is that?"

Themes	Clarifying Comments/Questions

is driven by the fear of what it is they don't remember or a fantasy that once they remember everything, they will be well.

Different styles of remembering

Some group members may remember only parts of their traumatic experiences, while others may remember the events in detail but not the feelings that go along with the events. Still others may have feelings that they are unable to link with the events. Often survivors become anxious about the ways they remember their experiences because the splintered fashion in which they remember makes them question whether or not the trauma really happened.

Leaders can help group members realize that these are all forms of remembering that are common in trauma survivors. The leader can emphasize the point that traumatic memories seem to be encoded differently from ordinary memories, and that this is the reason they are often remembered in a splintered fashion. Leaders might help members talk about their doubts, "Has anyone else felt this way? That because they can only remember parts of their traumatic experiences they must not be true?"

Another frequent theme is "What I remember about my childhood is bad enough. What about the things I don't remember? That's what scares me."

Remembering and dissociation

Group members will present with different ways that dissociation affects how they remember their histories. Some members may start to become dissociated when they remember their traumatic experiences (e.g., curl up in a ball and talk in a childlike voice when recounting their abuse). Group members often find their tendency to dissociate to be shameful and, as a result, they hide it in their everyday lives.

The leader can point out that there are many forms of dissociation, and that often these may have developed spontaneously as ways of coping with the trauma while it was occurring, but that they feel out of control now. Group members often know a great deal about dissociation. The leader might ask, "Can anyone explain what she thinks of as dissociation?"; "Why do you think trauma survivors dissociate?"

Sharing memories in a safe place

At some point, trauma work inevitably involves processing the trauma. This may be done in individual or group therapy and may involve sharing with friends and family when the survivor is ready. Many survivors have had negative experiences sharing their histories and need to learn when it is safe to do so and when it is not.

The leader might say, "Many times survivors share their traumatic experiences with someone, only to have them rejected or to be told they were lying or even told 'What's the big deal?' As a result, they don't share these experiences with anyone. Has any of you had positive experiences sharing your trauma histories—maybe with a therapist or close friend? What made those experiences positive?" The leader might also help members differentiate when it is safe to share the trauma and when it is not. "How do you know that it is safe to share your history with someone?" The point should be made that one way to know if someone is safe is to share

Themes	Clarifying Comments/Questions
	a little information with another person first, "test the waters," and then share a little more if the member gets the response she would like.
Self-care and remembering	Leaders should make the connection between self-care and remembering. In order to cope with the feelings that arise around remembering, group members need to take care of themselves physically and emotionally through exercising, eating well, and developing social supports. Leaders might ask members, "Are there things you do for yourself that help you when you are having memories?"

Additional suggestions frequently offered in this session are:

1. A grounding exercise when a member suffers from nightmares. Group leaders can suggest that she get out of bed, if she can, and walk to the bathroom. They direct her to look at her hands: "Look at them and remind yourself: these are the hands of an adult, not a child. I am safe." Then she can take turns washing her face with warm and cold water. The temperature changes can be regulating, and the intentionality of the behavior can be helpful in grounding.
2. A self-talk exercise to cope with flashbacks. Group leaders often share the example of a former group member who shared that when she had a flashback, she would mimic the emergency testing mechanism she heard on the radio, and say to herself, "This is a test of the trauma system. This is just a test. I'm safe."

Session 5: Shame and Self-Blame

The topics in sessions 4–8 (Remembering, Shame and Self-Blame, Self-Compassion, Anger, and Self-Image/Body Image) are among the most evocative and potentially distressing sessions in this group. It is for this reason that these topics are addressed in the middle sessions of the group, once clients have settled into the group and are more comfortable with the structure and with each other. They are not left for the last sessions because it is important that the group ends on a note of optimism and containment.

Shame is a difficult topic for many people because talking about shame often engenders feelings of shame. Shame can be a self-reinforcing emotion: people can be ashamed of feeling ashamed. Group leaders should mention this fact during the beginning of the session, so that these feelings do not take members by surprise. Group leaders can help prevent members from becoming immersed in shameful feelings by directing the discussion toward more positive topics, such as successful ways of coping with shame and ways members have found to differentiate between ordinary and destructive shame. By talking about their shame, group members begin to learn that destructive shame is a consequence of being traumatized. We have found that in this session members often discuss and reflect on current events and the impact of the societal blaming of victims that magnifies their sense of shame, as in the following table.

Themes	Clarifying Comments/Questions
Differentiating between guilt and destructive shame Survivors often have difficulty distinguishing between the feeling that they did something bad or made a mistake (guilt) and the feelings that they themselves are bad and broken (destructive shame).	Leaders should help group members begin to make distinctions between destructive shame and guilt. "Can people think of times when they've recently felt bad about something? Let's look at that. Was that about something you did or a feeling that you yourself were bad?" An example of this is a survivor who did something wrong at work and, instead of saying to herself, "I did something wrong. I need to fix it," she said to herself, "I screwed up again of course. I'm worthless." Destructive shame occurs when we feel totally worthless, dirty or disgusting, and unworthy of care or respect.
The connection between destructive shame and a trauma history Group members may not make connections between their trauma histories and their destructive shame. One survivor would repeatedly say, "Something must have been terribly wrong with me for my mother to treat me like that" and did not connect this belief about herself to her abuse history.	If members do not make a connection between their histories and destructive shame, leaders should comment on the connection. "Shame is often connected to the feeling that you are hiding something bad or toxic. As a child, many of you might have kept secrets about your abuse that over time grew into this feeling of shame. Now you may still feel as if there is something terrible about you that you are hiding from others. You may feel that if others really knew you they would loathe you and shun you." Or "Shame can develop if you got the message that the abuse you received was what you deserved. It might have been easier to blame yourself for being abused than your parents for abusing you." In recent groups, members have said, "I thought I had a quality that made good men want to do bad things" and "In my family, as the child, whatever you did, you did wrong."
Shame and anger Although anger is covered in another session, members may talk about how it is easier to feel shame than to feel anger. Some members find the strength of their anger scares them. In addition, members may identify being angry with being like their perpetrators—making it difficult to feel angry without feeling both ashamed and guilty. Being angry	Leaders may want to be explicit about possible connections between shame and anger. In a recent group, a member said, "I wake up every day and I'm like 'Damn it, I'm still me.' And I feel angry about it and wish I wasn't. I have to step back and remind myself not everyone has had these bad experiences, that's why they're not as messed up as me." It is important that leaders remind the group that there will be another session devoted entirely to anger. The goal of this group is to stay with shame as a primary focus. "One way we can understand shame is that when the abuse was happening it may have been safer to feel

Themes	Clarifying Comments/Questions
may also mean shifting blame from themselves to their perpetrators, and this is complicated for many survivors. For example, one member talked about how if someone gave her any sort of critical feedback, the criticism would tap into her feelings of destructive shame, and she would immediately lash out at the person. This response would then make her feel more ashamed because her behavior was often inappropriate.	ashamed than to feel angry. Can anyone talk about why this might be true?" This intervention is aimed at helping the group members learn from one another. "For those of you who have gotten past the place of feeling that you were responsible for what happened, can you share what helps you be there?"

Shame and self-blame and gender issues
 	
We have found that many trauma survivors feel a sense of shame about their gender and gender identity.
	Male survivors will often say, "If I was sexually abused, I'm not really a man. I'm passive so that's definitely not manly."
	
	   Group members may have been told, explicitly or implicitly, that their gender was bad. Male survivors frequently comment, "I never wanted to be my father. But my whole life I was told, 'You're just like your father, all men are made that way, to be alcoholics and wife beaters.'" Women have said, "I grew up thinking women are worthless because my mother was beaten and couldn't stop it, and I was abused and couldn't stop it. There's something about us being weaker. That's why I got my tubes tied."
	
	   Still others have a counterphobic reaction to feeling ashamed and powerless about these gendered dynamics: "If people could always just take whatever they wanted, I may as well make money at this by hustling with my body."
	
	   Still others express shame at looking female and talk about how they wear only bulky clothes for self-protection: "If I don't look like a woman, men won't look at me."
	
	   In response to these comments, leaders should make the connection between shame and gender identity and discuss how this is a function of how people internalize what happened to them. For example, a leader in one group said, "It is difficult identifying with your gender if you see your gender being treated badly or behaving badly. For example, if your mother is battered, you learn something negative about what it means to be a woman. People may ascribe words like *strong* and *weak* to *men* and *women*."

Shame and self-blame result from seeing oneself as a willing participant rather than a victim.	Leaders might say, "Sometimes people feel shame because they see themselves as participants in their abuse rather than as victims. Have people struggled with that? Can you

Themes	Clarifying Comments/Questions
Members might feel that they were complicit in their abuse or victimization for many reasons. They might have been told they wanted the abuse; they might have enjoyed the attention from the abuse; their bodies may have responded with pleasure to sexual stimulation; they might have played along with the perpetrator in order to survive. Beliefs about being a participant rather than a victim are often deeply rooted.	say more about that?" Some group members have found it helpful when leaders encouraged them to evaluate their participation in their abuse objectively. Another intervention that works well here is to ask members, "For those of you who were abused in childhood, how tall were you at the time?" As members raise their hands, ask them to look around the room and say, "Does anyone think someone that young, that small, could be responsible for abuse?"
	Asking members to visualize themselves as children can be effective, particularly because so many trauma survivors have a sense of themselves as much bigger and more capable than they in fact were.
	If a member was victimized in adulthood, we have found it helpful to have her think about her experience happening to someone she knows and cares about—for example, a sibling or a friend—and ask, "Would I hold this person responsible for what happened to her?"
	Finally, leaders should drive the point home that, even if a person did something that showed poor judgment and made her vulnerable—(e.g., got drunk in a bar with strangers), she still did not deserve to be victimized. An example that might be appropriate here is: "If you carelessly left your car on the street unlocked with the keys in the ignition, would someone have the right to steal your car?"
	It is important to emphasize that responsibility for abuse or assault always lies with the perpetrator.
Ways of challenging destructive shame	Leaders should end the session on a hopeful note, talking about ways to combat shame, emphasizing in particular that caring relationships with others are a particularly powerful antidote to shame. To enlist the group members in this exercise, leaders might ask, "Has anyone found anything that was helpful in challenging destructive shame?" Leaders can also call attention to particular interactive moments in the group and ask whether positive regard from others about something a member has shared helped detoxify the feelings of shame. Strategies can include directly challenging shame-filled thoughts by actively caring for oneself or doing something to help others. There are several other suggestions in the worksheet.

Session 6: Compassion

The session on compassion was not one of the original sessions in the group. It evolved organically and grew to be an important topic that followed naturally from discussions of shame and self-blame. In addition to the themes addressed in the worksheet, the issues presented in the following table also tend to come up in this session.

Themes	Clarifying Comments/Questions
"It is easier to feel compassion for others, including other group members, than myself." Many trauma survivors struggle with self-compassion because this feeling does not come naturally to them.	"Why are you afraid of having compassion for yourself? What comes up when you think about this?" Members often say, "I did not have kind role models and was not allowed to be kind or gentle to myself in any way growing up." Other examples from recent groups are: "I can only feel that for others. I have third-party compassion. I watch TV shows with the kids and I cry like a baby. I call it third-party grieving" and "Because of you all in the group, I maybe don't have compassion yet, but I have acceptance and understanding. Compassion means accepting the pain, and I'm not there yet."
The only way to have gotten through a traumatic event is to use "tough talk"—"Stop crying, stop feeling sorry for yourself."	Leaders may ask, "Can people volunteer what sort of self-talk comes up?" Members often say, "I'm not good enough," or "I don't feel human enough to have compassion for myself," or "I don't deserve to feel compassion." Leaders can then ask, "What are some responses you can say back to that part of yourself?"
The relationship between perfectionism and compassion	"If I'm not going to do 100%, I'm not going to do it at all." Many trauma survivors talk about how immobilizing this attitude can be for any efforts they make. This discussion can be very validating. A group member recently said, "It feels so good to listen to people and be like 'Yeah, me too' because I'm never with people who get it."
The relationship between self-blame and compassion	When trauma is caused by human cruelty, the effects are worse and last longer than trauma caused by "acts of God." Part of the reason is because survivors blame themselves for being victimized. Leaders may say, "If you survived a tsunami, you wouldn't tell yourself, I caused the tsunami. But the reason you struggle with compassion is because it was not a tsunami, it was a person, usually a person you trusted."

A powerful intervention in this group is to have the members go around and read the list of personal rights listed in the worksheet. This is one of the few times they read from the worksheet. During the closing check-in, leaders ask the members to look at the list of personal rights again and think about which one they would like to pay attention to in the coming week. This is what we call an "intentionality prompt" in the group—encouraging members to feel a sense of intention in their lives.

Session 7: Anger

Survivors' problems with anger tend to oscillate between extremes. On the one hand, survivors may experience intense rage that they have difficulty managing and, on the other hand, they may have difficulty getting angry at anyone—even the perpetrator. When they do get angry, they often experience intense self-loathing because anger makes them feel identified with a perpetrator and feel out of control. This is an extremely evocative session and the following table presents some of the common themes.

Themes	Clarifying Comments/Questions
Anger as a basic human emotion Leaders may say, "Because so often the people who abused survivors were angry when they did so, survivors often are afraid of anger and view it as something bad. When they feel anger, they may experience an identification with the perpetrator and therefore may deny their anger. Survivors have rarely had role models for handling anger appropriately."	Leaders should emphasize that anger is a feeling that everyone has at one time or another and that anger, when acknowledged, can give us useful information about relationships. Leaders should also address members' conflicts around anger. For example, "Some survivors have had a hard time feeling angry because their anger is so powerful that it scares them. Others have trouble feeling grief or sadness and have an easier time being angry. Susan, I see you nodding. What part of what I said makes sense to you?" Recent comments from groups include "If I let anger start, it just lets in the whole cycle of self-hatred. If you can picture driving through a fire, that was me for like a year. I wanted the whole world to hurt as much as I did, if I could have, I would have set fire to the world. But then it would make me feel even more angry because I'd wake up and be like, I'm terrible." Another example is "I would rather be angry than sad; at least anger is an awake emotion; crying on the floor doesn't accomplish anything."
The distinction between constructive and destructive anger	Leaders should make the distinction between the two types of anger and encourage members to give examples of each one. Survivors often have many experiences of destructive anger, for instance, when their parents used to beat them for making a mistake, but fewer examples of constructive anger. Leaders might say, "Has anyone had good experiences expressing their anger?" or "Has anyone had the experience of having their anger alert them when something was wrong in a relationship?" In a recent group, a member said, "If you're getting angry on behalf of someone else, it's constructive anger, it's halfway there. You can learn to speak up for others in ways we can't yet for ourselves."

Themes	Clarifying Comments/Questions
	Leaders should also emphasize that members should take pride in themselves for expressing anger constructively— even if they do not get the response they want from the other person. Righteous anger can also bring people together to resist injustice.
The connection between experiences of anger and survivors' comfort level in recognizing it, expressing it, and/or receiving it If survivors have experienced anger only as violent, then they may be uncomfortable even recognizing their own anger, let alone expressing it. If they feel that someone is angry with them, the feeling may send them into a panic because they may unconsciously fear the anger will lead to violence.	"Often people have difficulty dealing with anger because of negative experiences with it when they were growing up. Has anyone here made sense of her difficulties dealing with anger now in light of her past?" If group members have difficulty with this concept, leaders might want to be more explicit: "For example, in one group, a woman talked about how she would be terrified anytime she thought anyone was mad at her. Eventually, she recognized that in her head she linked anger with being beaten and anticipated that anyone who was angry at her would physically harm her."
Issues with anger "that come out of nowhere" Often survivors may be angry but aren't sure why. Or they may be angry about everything, but not be able to identify the particulars. This anger may be related to past losses and trauma and have less to do with what is going on in their current lives.	Leaders might raise this issue by saying, "Sometimes people just feel angry and don't really know why. Or they find their anger comes out at people who don't really deserve it, perhaps a spouse or a child. Does this sound familiar to anyone?" If this is an issue for group members, leaders may initiate a discussion on how to handle disproportionate anger. "Has anyone found ways that help deal with this kind of anger?" In the past, group members have found stress-reduction techniques helpful with anger. Also, some survivors have been able to identify and avoid situations that increase their general level of irritability.
"If I allow myself to feel angry, I'll get out of control."	Leaders may say, "It is important to remember that anger is a feeling, not necessarily something that leads to action. This can help anger feel less scary and overwhelming. In fact, letting yourself know you're angry with someone but choosing not to express it, and being able to hold that feeling yourself, can be an important experience, as it enables you both to own your feelings and also to feel a sense of control over them." This can lead to a deeply emotional experience for group members. In recent groups, members said, "Anger is ugly and nasty so as 'people pleasers' it feels like what's the point, it won't change anything," and "If people see angry me, they're like 'Whoa!' It changes their perception of

Themes	Clarifying Comments/Questions
	me. I've spent my whole life being like 'what can I do to help you?'"
The need to find safe ways to express anger	Leaders should end the session with a discussion of helpful ways to manage anger. "What would healthy anger look like?" "What about times when you can't address your anger at the people you are angry with because they are not available or because it's too dangerous? What do you do with those feelings?" Members can then give examples of ways to work with their anger and find sublimated ways to express it: artistically, physically (e.g., running, furious housecleaning), or comically.
	It can be important here for leaders to address what a sensory experience anger is for most people. Anger is often held in the body, felt in the stomach, and shown in the redness of the face and the gritting of teeth. Group leaders may say, "When you admit you're angry, it's important to breathe and say to yourself, 'This is anger.' Claim it so that you don't turn it inward or act impulsively." Physical ways of coping, such as a quick walk, can be very helpful here.

At times, this discussion can lead to conflict between group members. As an example, one member tried to give advice to another regarding her anger by saying, "You won't feel so angry if you are around safe people. You need to put yourself in safe and comfortable situations." The other member responded by saying, "You're deluding yourself if you think there's such a thing as a safe place." In keeping with the group philosophy of education and connection, rather than the processing of group dynamics, the leaders do not directly address the anger between members. It is generally more helpful to make a cognitive intervention such as "Beliefs about safety and relationships can come from so many places. Often they are part of a continuum." Leaders can also explain that people who give advice are really trying to be helpful, but what works for one person may not work for another. They can also suggest that rather than telling others what they ought to do, group members can simply share what works for them, along with their hope that others will find their suggestions helpful. This general principle holds for all topics, but is particularly true for the discussion of anger.

Session 8: Self-Image/Body Image

We have found that this topic is very emotional for group members. For women, the topic often brings up fears of being unattractive, ambivalence about their femininity, and, sometimes, outright hatred of their bodies. For men, this topic raises ambivalent feelings about their masculinity. If a man has been abused by another man, he may have conflicts about what it means to be a man, wondering whether being masculine means being an abuser.

Men have also acknowledged being self-conscious about their bodies. Male survivors often express deep conflicts about feeling themselves in their bodies, particularly if their perpetrators were men, and express concerns about their gender identification with the aggressor. Additional themes are addressed in the following table.

Themes	Clarifying Comments/Questions
How our family environment affects our body image	Leaders can help members think about how familial attitudes about their bodies and sexuality have influenced their body image. "After reading the Section 8 worksheet, can anyone think of examples of what messages they were given when they were children about their bodies? How did these messages affect you?"
How our culture affects our body image	The way in which our culture affects body image is a topic that raises a great deal of discussion among group members. A question as simple as "Does anyone have any ideas about how culture has affected her body image?" Leaders can prompt the discussion by using examples, such as the Barbie doll, the extremely thin models in magazines, and so on. For all-male or coed groups, leaders should encourage members to think about how cultural stereotypes affect men. For example, how does the boy who is not athletic feel about his body?
How trauma affects our body image	After reading the third paragraph of the worksheet, leaders should encourage members to think about how their traumatic experiences have affected their feelings about their bodies. Using the examples in the handout, leaders can ask, "These are just some ways in which being traumatized affects how we relate to our bodies. Do any of these sound familiar to anyone? Jo, you are nodding, what resonates with you?"
The relationship between self-care and body image	For survivors who so often express their distress through harming their bodies, learning to care for their bodies is a crucial step in recovery. Leaders should raise the point that members can develop a positive body image by caring for their bodies. Often survivors find that as they start caring for their bodies, they feel better about themselves, and this in turn creates a virtuous cycle. "Often members have talked about a relationship between how they care for their bodies and how they feel about themselves. Does this sound familiar to anyone?"
New ways of taking care of our bodies	Leaders should end discussion of the topic by having members think about the steps they have taken to care for their bodies and new things they can try. Some examples include getting more rest, eating more vegetables, exercising regularly, practicing

Themes	Clarifying Comments/Questions
	relaxation, being consistent with personal hygiene, going to the doctor or dentist for regular checkups, and so forth.
Sex and body image Sex and struggles with sexuality are a frequent discussion point in this group. It is important for leaders to normalize this topic and talk about how it goes beyond trauma and trauma recovery.	Leaders may say, "Most of us think sex comes easily to other people. But everyone struggles with sexuality. Sex is about vulnerability. When you have sex with a partner, you are being asked to feel things in those parts of your body that are most often associated with trauma memories. How can you ground yourself to remind yourself that this is the present and not the past when you are having flashbacks during sex? How can you alert your partner to what you are feeling, so that he or she can share in making sex in the present a very different experience from what you suffered in the past?" Another frequent theme is members' sense that they only have sex for someone else or to make another person happy. A frequent statement is "I don't know how sex can even be possible if I'm not drunk to get me through it." Explain to the group that sex freely chosen, with a caring partner, can be altogether different from coerced sex, an experience of pleasure rather than of humiliation.
Sexual orientation and trauma Many survivors, particularly men who identify as gay, discuss their complicated feelings about being a gay man. We have seen people express internalized homophobia in the group or express how homophobia has affected them, for example: "I know I'm not gay because I was abused. Everyone's told me this. But how come I prefer a male body? Intellectually I understand it's not because I was abused by a man, but a part of me wonders and has a lot of self-hatred."	It is really important here for leaders to jump in directly and unambiguously. This is another way in which this group differs from a psychodynamic or process group. The group leader may say, "I don't want to dismiss your feelings at all, but I do want you all to know that there is a lot of research about this, and the results are very clear: abuse does not 'cause' people to be gay or bisexual. If it did, there would be an awful lot more gay people because, as we all know, child abuse is very common. Most abuse survivors are heterosexual. And no, the abuse didn't cause them to be heterosexual, either." "Abuse can engender feelings of self-hatred and self-blame, as we talked about earlier, which can include feeling that one's sexual orientation is a sign of being damaged."

Session 9: Relationships

Leaders should be sure to remind members that this is the second to last group session. Since the topic is relationships, this session offers a time for members to consider their relationships with one another and anticipate the loss that will occur when the group ends. Session 3 (Trust) focused on members learning to trust themselves. This session focuses on how to build trust with others and deepen relationships.

Survivors are often acutely aware of how their histories negatively affect their current relationships. Many will say, "In relationships, I'm always waiting for the other shoe to drop. Always waiting to be judged or abandoned or betrayed or fired," or "It's the sense always that I have a scarlet letter." Many will talk about the benefit of having one's guard up, saying, "It's too scary to be vulnerable." Additional themes are provided in the following table.

Themes	Clarifying Comments/Questions
The effect of trauma on relationships Some survivors engage in relationships in which they are revictimized; others avoid relationships at all costs.	Leaders can ask, "How do you see your histories affecting your current relationships?" If members are slow to make the connection, leaders can give examples. Relationships with people in authority in which the other person has more power—bosses, doctors, or therapists—are often problematic for trauma survivors. If one has been abused or exploited in the past, it is hard to trust that power will be used fairly and responsibly. Because of their histories, some members may misinterpret the behavior of others or may react in an extreme way. For example, a survivor might attribute her boss's bad mood to something she has done when, in fact, her boss is upset about something that has nothing to do with her. Or a male survivor whose partner is angry with him may feel so threatened that he might lash out at her or storm out of the apartment rather than talk it out.
How to risk connections and find mutuality	Members will say, "I don't know whether I have the skills to pick someone good. I've become involved with bad guys so much that either everyone is a bad guy in the world or I have bad radar. How do I know if someone is trustworthy?" Leaders might ask, "How have others learned to let people in?"; "Does anyone have an example of how she judged whether another person was trustworthy?"
Connections to others feel limited, or the survivor is always in the same role	Members will say, "Either you're the caretaker or the problem solver or the needy person. You don't feel good about how you show up, how the other person shows up" or "When I'm with people who are more screwed up than me, or someone I am worried about, I'm the savior. It feels good to focus on someone else." A discussion of this common pattern can feel detoxifying to members. Leaders can also ask, "Does anyone have an example of how she changed a relationship to make it feel less confining and more authentic?"

Themes	Clarifying Comments/Questions
Strategies for better relationships	Leaders should end the session by discussing ways members can improve their relationships. Some strategies might be learning to share one's history appropriately, asking for clarification if one is confused about something, not making assumptions, speaking up if someone has done something offensive.

If the group members have made strong connections to one another, the leaders might use examples of how trust has developed within the group to illustrate the process of building relationships. For example, the leader might say, "Trust builds slowly over time. In the first group, none of you knew each other and therefore of course you didn't really trust each other. You only shared a little of yourselves. Over time, you have developed some trust in each other and shared some very personal stories." These observations may encourage members to talk about how they find it easier to trust one another than people in other areas of their lives and why that might be true.

Part of the closing round is used to prepare for the last session. The leaders may say:

"Next week will be our last session. We are going to make sure we have enough time to say good-bye to one another. We will have a worksheet available, but we may not get through it. You can take it home to look over after you leave. The group leaders will go around and give some feedback to each of you about your progress since our first meeting. There will also be time for each of you to give feedback to the others. You can feel free to say something if you wish, but you don't have to."

Session 10: Making Meaning of the Past and the Process of Recovery

The last session needs to accomplish a number of tasks, which include reviewing what the group has accomplished, saying good-bye to each member and, as time permits, reviewing and discussing the final worksheet. The group in many ways follows the standard session structure, but saying good-bye and addressing the end of the group is the primary focus. Many group members have not had the experience of saying good-bye to people in a healthy and positive way. This group may provide their first such experience.

Session Outline

1. Review the day's schedule.
2. Introduce the opening check-in.
3. Introduce the relaxation exercise.
4. Conduct the group termination process.
5. Present and discuss the topic.
6. Conclude with a closing check-in.

Content of the Session

1. REVIEW THE DAY'S SCHEDULE

Leaders need to acknowledge from the start that this is the last meeting: "As I am sure everyone knows, this is the last session of the group. You have all accomplished a great deal in terms of your recovery by coming here each week and participating. We are going to save some time at the end of the meeting to reflect on our experience together."

2. INTRODUCE THE OPENING CHECK-IN

Leaders should introduce the opening check-in: "As we go around today and check in, people might want to reflect briefly on their experience in the group."

3. INTRODUCE THE RELAXATION EXERCISE

The leaders should use the relaxation exercise following the usual format. During the exercise, they may want to make statements about how members should feel good about themselves for completing the group and for taking the time to focus on their recovery.

4. CONDUCT THE GROUP TERMINATION PROCESS

This usually starts with the leaders making a comment to the group as a whole about the growth and resilience they have witnessed. They may say:

> "We want to say how much we have appreciated the opportunity to be here with you all. Many people are not really good at saying good-bye, and this can be true particularly when one has been traumatized. We want you to take credit for your hard work in the group and to say good-bye to the others in the room. This is a time to celebrate your accomplishment and feel proud of committing to and completing this important step in your recovery."

Members will often say at this point how they have avoided good-byes in the past.

The leaders should have previously made notes on the feedback they want to give to each member. Taking turns, they go around the room and speak to each person individually. As they complete giving their feedback, they can invite other members to add their thoughts. We have found that to be on the giving and receiving end of positive feedback is a very emotional experience. The leaders can normalize this experience by saying, "We appreciate that it's hard to be receiving or saying such positive things."

This process can take a major portion of the group time. Once it is complete, leaders can say, "Let's reflect a bit together and talk about making meaning of the past."

5. PRESENT AND DISCUSS THE TOPIC, AS ILLUSTRATED IN THE FOLLOWING TABLE

Themes	Clarifying Comments/Questions
"Why did this happen to me?" Many survivors, especially those who have suffered from chronic interpersonal violence, struggle with the question of why other people have hurt them.	After reading the first paragraph of the worksheet, the leaders can stop and ask, "What are your thoughts? Why do bad things happen? Do bad things happen to good people or do they happen to us because we deserve them?" This will often lead group members to talk about how they have, in the past, blamed themselves for their abuse.
The distinction between belief systems of childhood and adult understanding	After an initial discussion of some of the beliefs group members hold, leaders might find it helpful to ask, "Has anyone thought about where these beliefs might come from?" Often what we believe about why bad things happen is based on the belief system of our childhood. This belief system can include what we were taught (e.g., in church or in temple) and what we learned implicitly. By examining how our childhood experience affects our current beliefs we can begin to sort through our current beliefs, reject those that are unhelpful or damaging, and retain those that are healthier.
Both children and adults who have been traumatized attempt to find ways to make meaning of the experience. This often involves asking, "What did I do to deserve this?" A survivor who answers this question by blaming herself (e.g., "I was abused because I am worthless, stupid, ugly"), can sustain long-lasting damage to her self-esteem. However, this type of self-blame may serve many adaptive functions: it enables the survivor to avoid being angry at the perpetrator and to feel some illusion of control over the trauma ("If I am very, very good, it may not happen again").	After reading the third paragraph of the handout, leaders may want to ask clients about how they made sense of their abuse in the past and how they make sense of it now.

Themes	Clarifying Comments/Questions
Barriers to changing beliefs Self-blaming beliefs are often hard to change because they serve a protective function. For example, if an adult woman lets go of the belief that she was raped on a date because she was too flirtatious and replaces it with the belief that the rape was the choice of the perpetrator and had little to do with her behavior, she has to face the possibility that no matter how she behaves, she is at risk for being raped. In some ways, it may be more comforting for her to believe that she was raped because she was flirtatious; then she can tell herself, "If I am not flirtatious, I will not be raped." By clinging to this belief, she gains some illusion of control.	Leaders can encourage group members to examine what stands in their way of letting go of their damaging beliefs. "So now as an adult, you know intellectually that your being abused was not caused by your being bad, but why do you think part of you still believes this?" To survivors of adult trauma, leaders might ask, "Although you know intellectually that it wasn't your fault you were assaulted, why does part of you still blame yourself? What is stopping you from putting full blame on the assailant?"
What does recovery look like? Adult survivors, particularly those who have suffered from prolonged and repeated childhood trauma, often don't know what it might be like to recover.	Leaders should ask group members to talk about what recovery means to them. "Has anyone thought about what it might be like to move beyond this?" If members don't respond, the leader might ask, "Do some of you struggle with the feeling that recovery is elusive? That it is far away, not attainable?" Members may bring up unrealistic notions, such as "Recovery means to forget the trauma," or unattainable notions, such as "When I'm recovered I'll never feel bad again." Leaders can share these notions with the rest of the group: "Do other people believe that to recover means you have to forgive and forget?" Often the group members will question each other's assumptions.
Difference in recovery for childhood versus adult trauma survivors	One leader explained this difference as follows: "If someone has had a pretty good life and then suffers a single traumatic event in adulthood, recovery might mean getting back to her previous level of functioning. For someone else, who has had many traumatic experiences from early on in life, recovery means learning many things that she never had a chance to learn as a child. The recovery process will include developing self-respect and a sense of personal agency and learning how to be in relationships of mutuality."

Themes	Clarifying Comments/Questions
Recovery as a process	Leaders should emphasize that recovery is a process and that all group members have made some strides in that process. One leader said, "Sometimes when it feels hopeless, you have to remember to take the long view. Look back and think of the gains you made in the past year. For those of you here, you might say, 'I've made progress because I can be in a group, while a year ago the thought of being in a group might have terrified me.' Recovery should not be seen as some unattainable ideal but as something that you are always moving toward." Leaders may choose to have group members give examples of ways in which they have made progress in their recoveries.
Specifics of recovery	Leaders should help group members define specifically what recovery looks like for themselves. This often leads to a review of the stages of recovery, starting with safety, then telling the story of the trauma, and finally making meaning of the experience. Group leaders can raise the point that these stages often overlap. For example, one member may be increasing her safety by becoming sober and may at the same time be making meaning of her history by working with abused children.
Finding a survivor mission	Leaders can explain that one way to transcend personal suffering is to join with others to change the social circumstances that foster violence. There are numerous examples of survivors who have done this; leaders can cite whatever examples seem most relevant. Leaders should end this topic on a hopeful note by having members think about what their survivor mission might be.

6. CONCLUDE WITH A CLOSING CHECK-IN

Leaders should start the final closing check-in by expressing some of their feelings about the group and what it has accomplished. For example:

> "Let me say that it really was a privilege to work with all of you over the past 10 weeks. I know it has been difficult at times, but you have all stuck with it, and your commitment made this a great group. I am sad to see you all go, but I am also proud of the progress you've made in your recovery and hopeful about what the future holds for you."

As members go around and check in for the final time, leaders will need to watch the time to make sure everyone gets a chance to say good-bye. Leaders should also explain that once the group ends, members are free to get together with one another socially if they wish, but that they should not feel obliged to socialize and they should not expect the kind of emotional intensity that they felt in the group. Rather, they would be well advised to meet for enjoyable activities or for projects of mutual interest. Leaders may leave the room once the last session is over, allowing those who wish to stay an extra few minutes to exchange contact information.

CONCLUSION

In the session-by-session guide in Chapters 3 and 4, we provide many concrete illustrations of the basic themes of the TIG: feeling empowered by information; overcoming the barriers of shame, secrecy, and isolation; and making unbearable pain and darkness feel more tolerable through connections with others. By breaking down the "nuts and bolts" of running the group and highlighting the common themes that emerge, we hope to capture some sense of the richness of the discussions that unfold. The progress reviews undertaken in the final group sessions instill confidence that trauma recovery can be expected as a reward of persistent effort and that it can be paced and manageable, rather than amorphous and overwhelming, as too often it feels to both clients and therapists. In the next chapter, we delve into some of the challenges involved in group leadership.

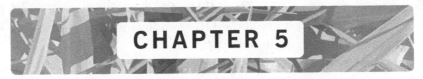

CHAPTER 5

Group Process
and Group Leadership

The TIG requires group leaders to attend to a multitude of tasks: managing time, providing education, assisting members to modulate their emotional distress, monitoring and containing the group process, and attending to the "arc" of the group, that is, the themes that emerge in beginning, middle, and ending sessions. Group leaders should therefore be able to draw on a solid conceptual knowledge of both complex trauma and group process, as well as a range of skills to manage acute trauma-related distress. Having access to consultants or supervisors is of utmost importance in supporting group leaders so that they can play the multifaceted roles required for successful implementation of the TIG.

REQUIRED KNOWLEDGE BASE FOR GROUP LEADERS

Leaders of the TIG should be appropriately trained and qualified mental health professionals (e.g., psychologists, social workers, psychiatrists, or psychiatric nurses) who have experience working with traumatized clients and facilitating therapy groups. They should be familiar with the clinical literature pertaining to the treatment of complex trauma and the particular population they serve, and they should also be conversant with the basics of the group process. We have outlined some of these areas along with suggested clinical sources in the table at the end of this chapter. A review of this material can serve as a form of self-assessment as clinicians gauge their sense of readiness to facilitate this group.

In addition to these areas of knowledge and skill, we consider it essential that clinicians who intend to conduct the TIG thoroughly read this treatment guide from start to finish *before* planning to start a group. They should then familiarize themselves with each chapter, so that they have a clear overview of the TIG from the initial screening process through each phase from beginning to conclusion.

The flexible content of this group does not lend itself to the sort of manual that prescribes word-for-word what clinicians should say. This treatment guide includes many verbatim examples of group leaders' explanations and interventions, but they are offered as suggestions only; clinicians both experienced and new to the model are strongly encouraged to use their own clinical judgment and their own unique communication styles as they assume the leadership role.

LEADER STANCE

Unlike the practice in a more traditionally psychodynamic group, in the TIG the leaders take an active and nonneutral stance. They express solidarity with victims of violence, they educate about trauma and its impact, and they intervene regularly throughout the group process. Group members have often experienced profound invalidation, shaming, and secrecy related to their experiences of trauma. Disclosures about trauma have often been met with dismissive or incredulous statements, such as "That was so long ago" or "I can't believe anyone would do that." In contrast, group leaders take a stance that is explicitly warm, compassionate, accepting, and validating.

For example, in a recent group, members engaged in a discussion about the #MeToo movement, in which numerous survivors of sexual harassment and abuse had spoken out publicly and had received a great deal of attention in the press. Group members reported that many of their coworkers and friends were critical of the campaign. One group member quoted an acquaintance who had stated with great authority, "Everyone is supposed to be considered innocent until proven guilty." She felt utterly at a loss to reply, and she related this feeling to her own history of being silenced and disbelieved as a child. At this point, the group leaders took a nonneutral stance. One leader said, "The idea is that people are supposed to be considered innocent until proven guilty has great merit, but unfortunately, sometimes it serves as a cover for societal denial about abuse. When we hear six similar stories of abuse by the same perpetrator, there is a credibility that is hard to ignore." This active educational stance conveys respect for group members and their experiences and facilitates engagement early in the group, when members are tentative and anxious about participating. It reassures group members that here their stories will not be discredited, not even with lofty principles.

Interventions highlighting the commonalities among group members help foster a sense of connection and cohesion. Members of this group often struggle with interpersonal relationships in their daily lives. Leaders encourage positive interactions and model empathic feedback between group members, which is often expressed in heartfelt and touching ways as the group progresses. Leaders intervene to minimize negative and potentially disruptive dynamics and to facilitate and elaborate on expression of empathy and support from members. The focus of the group is redirected from potential conflicts between the members toward the content of the worksheets or the discussions they are engendering.

Various individual dynamics are at play in the group room. Some clients have learned to relate to others by being "people pleasers" and trying to gratify others with their feedback, while others present as angry or shut down. In a traditional process group, leaders might ask someone to talk about what it's like to try to gratify others and where that need may come from. In this group, leaders may notice a person who tries to connect by pleasing others or tries to rally others through anger, but these are not dynamics that can be taken up directly in the group.

CO-LEADERSHIP

Co-leadership is the model we have generally used at the VOV Program, and we have found it to be valuable for many reasons. Because we are based in a teaching hospital, our model is designed to promote practical and hands-on skills building for the next generation of clinicians. Even in clinical settings that have no formal teaching component, however, co-leadership has many advantages. It allows leaders to attend to the needs of what can be a large group; if a member is having a panic attack or fleeing from the group, one leader can step out of the room with that person if necessary, while the other can continue conducting the group and keep the momentum going. Co-leadership also allows the co-leaders to model an egalitarian, mutually supportive relationship and increases the likelihood of group members speaking to one another rather than maintaining a focus on a single leader. It creates the opportunity for experienced leaders to train additional colleagues in the model, so that competency is disseminated within a clinical setting. Finally, co-leadership is a powerful antidote to the vicarious traumatization and burnout that can come from leading a TIG. For this reason, even though many settings have financial and human resource constraints, we recommend co-leadership because it can maintain staff morale and productivity over the long term. These groups can be and have been led successfully by one skilled leader, but in those cases it is important that the leader be offered support and consultation through some mechanism, such as private or program supervision.

When groups are co-led, it is important that group leaders also be aware of the dynamics and complexities involved in co-leadership (Delucia-Waack & Fauth, 2004). These dynamics are different for dyads in which one therapist has more experience and authority than the other, as in a training situation, compared with dyads in which the two leaders are peers (Rutan, Stone, & Shay, 2007). Where such differences exist, it is crucial that the dynamic of domination and subordination not be reenacted in the leadership pairing. Co-leaders should plan actively so that the student or the less-experienced clinician has a part to play in conducting each session, such as delivering the psychoeducational portion of the group. Leaders can also plan ahead for particular interventions, so that the less-experienced leader knows what she is responsible for saying in the group and a sense of mastery is promoted.

Regardless of their level of expertise, it is always helpful for group leaders to have regular access to a supervisor or consultant. Ideally, the supervisor should be a clinician who is experienced in conducting trauma treatment and group therapy. In any case, the supervisor should be familiar with this treatment approach and should read the manual thoroughly. Regular supervision or consultation has been identified as a key element in preventing secondary or vicarious traumatization among therapists (Salston & Figley, 2003; Vicarious Trauma Toolkit, n.d.). Therapeutic work with trauma survivors often poses unique challenges with regard to the therapist's countertransference. Supervision is one mechanism that can provide therapists with an opportunity to understand these reactions, so that they are not enacted to the detriment of the client or the group.

ARC OF THE GROUP

Early Sessions

Many members have never been in a successful group situation and are initially afraid to join a TIG. In early sessions, it is particularly important for group leaders to reflect the bravery and capability of group members, as well as to educate members about how participating in a group may in itself help them to improve their interpersonal relationships. When a group member participates in early sessions, a leader might say:

> "I'm so impressed that having just met these people, you can be so honest about your experience. I want all of you to stop for a moment and appreciate the fact that despite the anxiety you may be feeling, you all took a risk to come to the group to be known and to work on your healing. It is important to give yourself credit for your courage."

The group topics are arranged progressively, such that the more unifying topics come first. In the first session, group members often feel that they have finally met other people who can understand their experiences, and they may quickly idealize the group and its members. For this reason, they may not attend to the reality that the members can also have differences, and group leaders should be mindful to raise both similarities and differences in the early sessions in order to facilitate a less idealized or rushed bond between members. For example, when discussing the section in the first worksheet that addresses the relational impact of trauma, several group members may comment on feeling too dependent on others or indicate that they trust people more quickly than they should. A group leader might then ask, "Are there people here who go to the other extreme and who won't let anyone in? Can someone speak to why that might also be the outgrowth of trauma?"

In early sessions of the TIG, members primarily express the sense of validation they feel in not being alone in their traumatic experience, and group leaders echo this observation by saying that the group is intended to provide the kind of support they have always deserved. In a recent group, a client said, "I went home after the group and I just tried to feel good about who I am. When I heard other people say they struggle with the things that I get down on myself about every day, it made me feel less crazy and messed up."

Middle Sessions

During the middle sessions of the group, members become more comfortable being authentic with each other and having more moments of direct connection and support. Group leaders can often begin to use fewer interventions aimed at facilitating connection between members and more interventions that reflect and honor the growing connections they see developing. As they start to know group members more multidimensionally, the leaders continue to attend to members' resilience by reflecting on their capabilities, the steps they have taken to address trauma-related difficulties, and the progress they have made.

As the group continues, members have a better understanding of the ground rules about remaining focused on the present, and are less likely to share graphic details of their trauma histories in ways that are not appropriate. However, as the group feels more intimate, members will often share particular parts of their history that they might otherwise keep secret, feeling confident that they will not be shamed. For example, one group member shared the fact that she was HIV positive, a legacy of her heroin addiction. Another shared the fact that she had been forced into prostitution as a teenager. We have found that in a well-run group members will be unfailingly supportive and respectful of the confidences with which they have been entrusted. Many tears will be shed, but there will also be moments of genuine shared laughter.

Final Sessions

In the final sessions of the group, members are often worried about what they will do without the group. This is an opportunity to discuss how they can use some of the relational skills they may have learned in the group to form or improve relationships outside of a therapeutic context. For example, a group leader might comment, "David, you've always said you don't know how to relate to people. Now you see that not only can you relate to people, but also that they're very drawn to you. Can you see using that in other relationships?"

Leaders can also review options for members to participate in other forms of psychotherapy, including other trauma groups if they are available. Some members may wish to repeat the TIG, especially if they have only just begun to participate actively in the later sessions. We have had a number of clients who joined a second group and became much more engaged the second time around. Some members at the conclusion of this group may feel ready to embark upon a trauma-focused group, in which they will have the opportunity to speak about their histories in more depth.

When the group goes well, in the last session, leaders often feel that they have helped members navigate a developmental challenge of healing: to be able to tolerate being in a room with other people and to make themselves known and risk being seen. Honoring the healing of group members allows trainees and newer clinicians, particularly, to understand something of a trajectory of healing and the role of a therapist in that process. Clinicians observe the group members making connections, recognizing their skills in making those connections, and feeling pride in the abilities that they have gained. As therapists witness therapeutic skills being internalized, they also share in the group's sense of pride.

COMMON CHALLENGES

The TIG's structure is designed to minimize conflicts between group members and to increase group cohesion. Nevertheless, clinical challenges can arise in the group. Here we present examples of some clinical situations that we encounter frequently. Group leaders are encouraged to bring the breadth of their clinical experience to bear on any of these examples. Our descriptions here are not meant to be the final word on how to handle these challenging situations. Instead, we offer some guidelines based on the structure and purpose of the group, as well as our clinical experience working with traumatized clients.

The Client Who Is Silent during the Group

This challenge often arises in the group's early stages. Parts of the group sessions, such as the opening and closing check-ins, are constructed so that everyone's voice is present in the room. All group members are asked to participate in these parts of the group. Leaders can also facilitate participation of all members in a number of other ways. They can initiate a go-round, which is especially useful when multiple members seem tentative about speaking. For example, in a discussion of safety, the first topic, the group leader might say, "Let's just take a moment and all pay attention to what it feels like to know that 90% of you didn't even have the idea of what safety meant until you were adults. Can we go around and each just say something about what feelings this is bringing up?"

Leaders can also call on a silent member with an open-ended question. For example, as the first worksheet on common reactions to trauma is being discussed, a leader might say, "Renee, which reactions on this list speak to your experience?" If a silent member is nodding in apparent sympathy or agreement with a member who is talking, the group leader might use this as an occasion to call on her. For example, a leader might say, "Joanne, I noticed you were nodding when Nina was talking. Can you say something about what you were thinking when you were nodding?"

The choice of intervention often depends on what leaders perceive to be the nature of the client's silence. On the one hand, silence might reflect a client's feelings of shame or inadequacy. In this case, encouragement by leaders is important to help the client counter these feelings and have the experience of contributing to the group. The leader should also make an effort in this situation to comment in an affirming way on the group member's participation in order to counter her all-too-likely self-criticism ("I never say the right thing. I should keep my mouth shut").

On the other hand, a client's silence might reflect either extreme hyperarousal or dissociation. When a client is in an altered state, asking her to contribute to the group discussion is not helpful. Rather, one of the group leaders might observe that the topic is "pretty emotional" and suggest taking a break for some deep breathing or stretching. Often at the outset, leaders will not understand the nature of a client's silence. Usually, the reason becomes clearer over time. If clients repeatedly pass during "go-round" interventions, the group leaders can ask them to stay after the session in order to gain a better understanding of what may be contributing to their silence.

The Client Who Monopolizes the Group

Occasionally, a group may contain a member who is using the group to address her or his own issues to a degree where it becomes overbearing. If the talkative person has an individual therapist, a group leader may attempt to contain her by stating something like "Colleen, it seems like this topic brings up a lot of issues for you. I'm sorry that we don't have time to address them all here. Could you bring them up in your individual therapy?" Leaders may also try to generalize the discussion by remarking that the talkative person has raised some important issues and ask her to listen to some comments and feedback from others. Still another option is for the leader to interrupt the monopolizing member by addressing a comment to another person. A leader might say, "Rita, you seemed to be responding to what Emily was saying. Can you say something about what you were thinking?"

The Member Who Discloses Too Much of Her Trauma History

Occasionally, early on in the course of the group, a member may begin to talk in graphic detail about her trauma history. If this happens, it is important that the group leaders intervene quickly before even more disclosure occurs. They must be careful not to shame the client, which usually can be done by validating what the client is saying, while also helping to redirect the disclosure to the impact of the trauma. For example, the group leader might say, "Carla, I'm just going to stop you for a second. I'm really glad you're relating to this topic, and I know you're talking about really painful things. I'm going to ask you now to tell us more about how you *feel* about what happened, rather than sharing any more details." Very occasionally, some members feel that they are being silenced by the request not to discuss details of their trauma histories. If this concern is raised, the leaders could review once again the rationale for the group's focus on the present. The leaders can also explain that the goal is not to silence anyone, but rather to create a safe and containing environment for everyone.

The Member Who Becomes Extremely Dissociated during the Group

Since dissociation is a common symptom in clients with trauma histories, the group leaders should be attentive to the level of dissociation group members may be experiencing. Attending to a group member who is dissociating can become an opportunity for learning and group sharing. Leaders can educate the group about dissociation by defining what dissociation is and why it occurs. The leaders might say something like this:

> "Dissociation is a way of coping with overwhelming feelings that often develops in childhood. Imagine a child who is being abused and does not have the power to get away from the situation. By 'spacing out,' leaving her body, or shutting off her feelings, the child can remove herself mentally from the situation and thereby protect herself. This ability to dissociate may be adaptive to a harsh environment early in life, but can be problematic later. Many of you in this room may, at times, find that you are 'spaced out,'

emotionally disconnected from what is going on around you. You might feel that you are observing what is going on from a great distance. Has anyone had that experience?"

Often, group members will nod or respond to this question. This provides the opportunity for the group leader to ask members to talk more about their experiences of dissociation.

The leader should then direct the discussion to helping the dissociated member identify what she finds useful in grounding herself. Other members can offer ideas they find helpful when they find themselves dissociating. Before leaving this topic, the leaders should establish a way of checking in with the dissociated member if she begins to dissociate in future meetings. Often this may mean a brief intervention, such as asking the member a simple question using her name. The leader might say, "Sam, can you share what you are thinking?"

The Member Who Wants to Leave the Room during the Group

This situation occurs rarely and is usually due to a client's feeling emotionally overwhelmed. The first step is for the leaders to determine whether they can help the client stay in the room and bring her feelings into the zone of tolerance. If this is not possible, ideally, one leader can leave with the client and spend a few minutes with her, helping her regulate her feelings so that she feels ready to return to the group. If the leader cannot calm the client within a few minutes, the leader should ensure that the client is safe, discuss what she plans to do after leaving the group, and suggest that she should call her individual therapist or a friend for support.

The Member Who Sees Her History as Essentially Different

Occasionally, a client will see her trauma story as different from and incompatible with that of others in the group. In these instances, the leaders can explain that even with different histories, trauma survivors often cope in similar ways. This provides a further opportunity for talking about common reactions to trauma and symptoms of PTSD. Group leaders should further reemphasize that the purpose of the group is not to review the particular circumstances of the trauma story, but rather to examine the many ways that trauma affects survivors. They can reflect the fact that many trauma survivors feel "different" from ordinary people and ask the group if others have experienced themselves as "different" because of their histories.

CHALLENGES FOR CLINICIANS

Working with traumatized patients generates predictable emotional traps for clinicians. Here we outline some of the common issues that arise for leaders when running the group.

The Experience of Vicarious Trauma

Both inexperienced and seasoned clinicians are vulnerable to vicarious traumatization, or emotional reactions resulting from exposure to the traumatic experiences of others. Leading trauma groups can cause clinicians to experience intrusive imagery related to their client's experiences, challenge their feelings of competency, and disrupt their feelings of safety in the world. Organizations have a responsibility to be aware of the likelihood of vicarious traumatization and should provide adequate supervision and support for their staff. For a useful toolkit for organizations and individuals, clinicians may consult the Vicarious Trauma Toolkit (n.d.), developed by the Office for Victims of Crime.

Countertransference Reactions

These unavoidable feelings are part of any therapeutic relationship, but trauma patients tend to evoke intense reactions in many therapists. For example, many therapists will feel helpless or inadequate with a dissociated patient who is mute or monosyllabic. Others may feel angry and frustrated; still others may feel extremely protective. If a clinician is herself a trauma survivor who coped by being mute as a child, she may overidentify with this client. Splitting among clinicians is particularly common with trauma patients. It is up to all clinicians to pay attention to what is a normative reaction to this work and which of their reactions are unique given their own experiences. Addressing countertransference reactions frankly and openly with colleagues is a critical step in providing high-quality treatment. Again, supervisory support is crucial for this reflective work.

Communication between Leaders

During group sessions, it can be a challenge for the group leaders to communicate. They often have different opinions about how they perceive clients and their personal dynamics and may have varying ideas about pacing. It is to be expected that co-leaders will not always see eye to eye. When two colleagues are running a group together, issues around competition may arise. When the group leaders are unequal in their experience, as in the case of a seasoned clinician and a student or beginner, unconscious idealization and fear may come to the fore. Conflict between leaders, when unresolved, can be damaging to the group process; one leader may "take over" to establish dominance, while the other may disengage "just to get through the group." This disengagement often compounds the experience of vicarious trauma. Successful resolution of the conflict can be a valuable aspect of learning to lead a group.

It takes a skillful supervisor to "hold" what is happening in the group and between the leaders. It is important that supervisors create a safe environment in which conflicts can be discussed openly. Most important, any conflict between co-leaders must be addressed outside the group, rather than enacted within it. When group leaders feel secure in their ability to deal with their own personal and interpersonal problems, they communicate this confidence to the group.

Having Compassion for One's Limitations as a Group Leader

There are many tasks to manage in this group, and it is inevitable that certain issues and dynamics get prioritized over others. Group leaders may sometimes miss or misread cues from clients. In a recent group, a leader did not recognize that the group member sitting next to her had pushed her chair back and was looking dissociated and disconnected. As the group leader it is often a challenge to say to oneself as you would say to clients: You did the best you could.

CONCLUSION

As we have noted throughout this book, the group leaders face myriad tasks in running a TIG: providing a holding environment, keeping the group "on topic," educating members, assisting members to modulate their emotional distress, monitoring and containing the group process, and attending to the "arc" of the group. It is in some ways more art than science. It is inevitable that group leaders, especially in their first experiences of running the group, will feel that too often they lose control of the group process, that they try interventions that fall flat, or that they are not able to get to everything they had planned. However, we encourage group leaders to exercise for themselves the same compassion they provide for the group members. What we have found, over the years, is that the group structure is sturdy and holds its own against small tempests. The presence, validation, and support of the other group members are ultimately the "therapeutic action" and soul of the group. It is a deeply gratifying experience to bear witness to the compassion and wisdom that develop in this group and to facilitate a growing sense of hope among group members, who are often just beginning trauma-focused treatment, and who leave the group with the sense that recovery is possible.

Suggested Group Leader Knowledge Base and Suggestions for Readings

Complex Trauma and Recovery

Complex Trauma
- Characteristics of complex trauma
- PTSD, dissociation, and other trauma-related disorders
- Impact of trauma on developmental capacities and attachment
- Neurobiological consequences of chronic trauma

The Recovery Process
- Stages of recovery
- Psychotherapy with trauma survivors
  - Addressing trauma-related symptoms
  - Enhancing affect modulation and interpersonal functioning
  - Countertransference and vicarious traumatization

Key References

Courtois, C. A., & Ford, J. D. (Eds.). (2009). *Treating complex traumatic stress disorders: An evidence-based guide.* New York: Guilford Press.

Foa, E. B., Keane, T. M., Friedman, M. J., & Cohen, J. A. (Eds.). (2009). *Effective treatments for PTSD: Practice guidelines from the International Society for Traumatic Stress Studies* (2nd ed.). New York: Guilford Press.

Harvey, M. R., & Tummala-Narra, P. (Eds.). (2007). *Sources and expressions of resiliency in trauma survivors: Ecological theory, multicultural practice.* Binghamton, NY: Haworth Maltreatment & Trauma Press.

Herman, J. L. (2015). *Trauma and recovery.* New York: Basic Books. (Original work published in 1992)

Saakvitne, K. W., Gamble, S., Pearlman, L. A., & Lev, B. T. (2000). *Risking connection: A training curriculum for working with survivors of childhood abuse.* Baltimore: Sidran Press.

Group Therapy

Group Therapy Basics
- Curative factors in group therapy
- Stages of group development
- Group dynamics
- Preparing patients for group therapy
- Change process in group psychotherapy

Special Considerations
- Characteristics and types of groups
- Special issues in time-limited group therapy
- Group therapy with trauma survivors

(continued)

Suggested Group Leader Knowledge Base and Suggestions for Readings *(continued)*

Key References

Bernard, H. S., & Mackenzie, K. R. (Eds.). (1994). *Basics of group psychotherapy.* New York: Guilford Press.

Brown, D., Reyes, S., Brown, B., & Gonzenbach, M. (2013). The effectiveness of group treatment for female adult incest survivors. *Journal of Child Sexual Abuse: Research, Treatment, and Program Innovations for Victims, Survivors, and Offenders, 22,* 143–152.

Delucia-Waack, J. L., Gerrity, D. A., Kalodner, C. R., & Riva, M. T. (Eds.). (2004). *Handbook of group counseling and psychotherapy.* Thousand Oaks, CA: Sage.

Klein, R. H., & Schermer, V. L. (Eds.). (2000). *Group psychotherapy for psychological trauma.* New York: Guilford Press.

Mendelsohn, M., Herman, J. L., Schatzow, E., Coco, M., Kallivayalil, D., & Levitan, J. (2011). *The Trauma Recovery Group: A guide for practitioners.* New York: Guilford Press.

Mendelsohn, M., Zachary, R., & Harney, P. (2007). Group therapy as an ecological bridge to new community for trauma survivors. *Journal of Aggression, Maltreatment and Trauma, 14*(1–2), 227–243.

Rutan, J. S., Stone, W. N., & Shay, J. J. (2007). *Psychodynamic group psychotherapy* (4th ed.). New York: Guilford Press.

Valerio, P., & Lepper, G. (2010). Change and process in short and long-term groups for survivors of sexual abuse. *Group Analysis, 43*(1), 31–49.

Yalom, I. D., & Leszcz, M. (2005). *The theory and practice of group psychotherapy* (5th ed.). New York: Perseus Books.

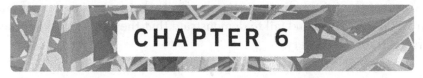

CHAPTER 6

Adaptations of the Trauma Information Group

"Would you tell me, please, which way I ought to go from here?"
"That depends a good deal on where you want to get to," said the Cat.
"I don't much care where—" said Alice.
"Then it doesn't matter which way you go," said the Cat.
—LEWIS CARROLL, *Alice's Adventures in Wonderland* (2011)

As has been referenced earlier, the TIG has proven to be a durable and adaptable group model for trauma survivors. In this chapter, we look more closely at these adaptations and also at the process of adaptation itself. Unlike Alice, who wanders aimlessly through Wonderland, when seeking a new direction for a group model it is important to know where you want to go, how you want to get there, why you want to go, and what you hope to achieve by going there.

Adaptations are essential and are part of the natural course of evolution if an organism is to survive. This is true for group models as well. A group is a living, vital organism. It requires skill and artistry on the part of the group leaders to balance the group's purpose, structure, philosophical underpinnings, and theory of change with the fluidity of each participant's current relationship to her trauma and the current context of her life. For this reason, treatment groups, even those that follow a manualized model, are inherently in a constant state of subtle adaptation and calibration.

More formal adaptations of group models are useful when the model, as it is structured, does not resonate with the population being served, the current context does not support the model, or the group leaders have new skills that they would like to integrate formally into the model. Additionally, we know that the group will not be effective if group members do not believe that the information presented reflects their experience, or if group leaders are insecure or ill-prepared and fail to demonstrate that they are steeped in the awareness of the course of trauma recovery.

THE PROCESS OF ADAPTATION

Although we have likened group models to living organisms, we may also consider the process of redesigning or adaptation of a group model as similar to the redesigning of a home. Our homes, though inanimate, are in a constant interplay with our changing needs. Our approach to life is reflected within them. Any of us who have attempted home repairs or renovations are familiar with the challenge of fitting our desires to the inherent limitations of our homes. We may yearn for more light, but the wall we wish to remove is a bearing wall, and removing it would leave us with a structurally unsound and unsafe home. However, as long as the structural integrity is maintained, changes are possible. An opening in the wall rather than its complete removal may bring in more natural light as well as produce the lifestyle we were seeking. It is in conversations with an architect or contractor that a design is based on the interplay between factors, such as expense, structural determinants, time, building codes, and so forth, and our aesthetic desires. Similarly, we may think of the group model as serving the function of a "home base," a structural "safe place" for group members. So, borrowing from the field of architecture and design, we want to identify the "bones" of the group model and to maintain its "bearing walls." For group models, the "bones and bearing walls" are the key theoretical constructs and principles and the structural elements that maintain the integrity of the group model and contribute to a safe and beneficial group setting.

THE PRINCIPLES OR "BEARING WALLS" OF THE TRAUMA INFORMATION GROUP

We described the trauma theory underlying the TIG in the previous chapters, so here we only briefly reiterate essential principles and recast them as the "bones and bearing walls" that contribute to the integrity of the model's structure. These include the following premises:

1. Safety in the group is based on predictability, reliability, and transparency. All aspects of the group process must reflect these qualities. This includes the structural framework (adherence to time parameters, group guidelines, and expectations), as well as clinical interventions.
2. Because interpersonal acts of violence take place in a familial and sociopolitical context, an ecological/contextual approach is required in order to understand the psychological impact of these acts. Because trauma causes a tear in one's social/relational fabric, the repair occurs relationally.

3. Relational repair occurs in part through education about the impact of trauma, as well as through the validation and normalization of the predictable reactions to traumatic events.

4. Recognition of domains of functioning allows for group members to appreciate their inherent resilient capabilities and to reframe symptoms as functional adaptations that can become maladaptive.

5. Recognition that suffering is universal, even though the experience of suffering is specific to the individual, promotes compassion for self and others.

6. Attention to the therapist processes, as well as to group processes, promotes the values of dignity and respect.

Combined with an understanding of group dynamics and group processes, these fundamental principles or "bearing walls" offer us a complex and nuanced understanding of the interplay of the fields of traumatic experience and determine how we craft our interventions.

ESSENTIAL ELEMENTS: THE "BONES" OF THE TRAUMA INFORMATION GROUP STRUCTURE

The "bones" of the TIG are found in its structural framework. This framework in the analogy we are using is supported by the "bearing walls." The three main elements of this structure are first, the settling-in period; second, the topic overview with facilitated discussion; and finally, the closing. Although there may be some variation within each of these elements, they are essential to the integrity of the group model and are not readily adaptable.

What Elements of the Group Model Are Adaptable?

We can use the ecological model developed by Harvey (1996) as a source for understanding the components that are variable and therefore more naturally adaptable. As identified, the ecological model looks at three broad categories that influence the response to a traumatic event: person, event, and environment (Harvey, 1996). If we transpose these categories to a group context, we can view "person" as the composition of the group (number of participants, homogeneous vs. heterogeneous group membership with respect to trauma histories, current functioning, cultural background, gender, age, language, etc.). We view "event" as the parameters of the group (duration of the group, frequency of meetings, length of sessions, intervals between sessions). Finally, we can view "environment" as the setting in which the group takes place (clinic, office, hospital, community), the setting in which the participants live (urban, rural, hospital), the fiscal constraints (insurance, fees, staffing, liability concerns), and the sociopolitical context in which the trauma(s) occurred and in which the group is being offered. These are the variables that may change over time and thereby determine the adaptations.

Why Adapt This Model?

As we mentioned in the beginning of this chapter, adaptations are useful when one is aware that the model, as structured, will not resonate predictably with the population being served, the current environmental context does not support the model, or the group leaders have new skills that they would like to integrate into the model in order to express their own professional creativity. When adapting a group model, it is important to retain its essence—the key theoretical constructs, principles, and essential elements—and to take into consideration the characteristics of the population being served. Of equal importance is articulating a theory of change in a way that explains why the model was adapted. Here we offer several examples of TIG adaptations that have been developed by staff at the VOV Program or colleagues at other agencies who worked closely with VOV staff.

PASSAGEWAYS: INCORPORATING CREATIVE ACTIVITIES

After several years of co-facilitating the TIG with Lois Glass, Barbara Hamm began to develop other group models that were influenced by her early training in child development and play therapy. This translated into bringing elements of play and creative interactions into the group process. This adaptation of the TIG kept the structure of the group—time frame, elements (settling in, topics, and closing)—and stayed true to an understanding of recovery from trauma that identifies predictability, transparency, and reliability. Group members were expected to be punctual, stay the entire time, and notify the group leaders of any absences. This was also true for the group facilitators. The provision of psychoinformation that emphasized the sociopolitical context of trauma and considered symptoms as adaptations was maintained as the foundational offering. The activities were paired to the topics and this foundational framework.

The adaptations followed Mildred Parten's (Parten & Newhall, 1943) *stages of play* therapy by introducing solitary, onlooker, parallel, associative, and cooperative play into the group process. Parton was an early observer of children's play and was one of the first to suggest that when children are at play they learn how to interact with others, how to cooperate, and how to share and to make friends. Since we know that traumas experienced early in life disrupt normal childhood developmental tasks, these skills are often underdeveloped in the adults we see who have childhood trauma histories. Parton identified the stages of play that are developmentally sequenced so that cooperative play, the culminating stage, brings together the skills drawn from all previous stages, enhancing the child's capabilities for social and group interactions (Parten & Newhall, 1943).

Each component of the group incorporated play activities paired to the topic of the week. Each session also incorporated a progression of five stages of play, which included using movement and physical interactions. When groups are organized around members sitting in a circle, people often take the same position week after week. They may choose to sit next to the facilitator or a "safe" group member. Their view from their seat is the same. While this arrangement offers predictability, one of the elements we referenced as essential, members' physical energy is often held in check and has little motoric opportunity for discharge or release. When learning is primarily verbal and auditory, those patients for whom these modalities of learning are not most easily accessible will sometimes be left behind, and it will take a skilled therapist to draw them out without invoking shame.

Movement was therefore introduced into each session, both to afford group members new perspectives in the room and to encourage them to take in information in multiple modalities. Movement was introduced in natural ways, such as reaching across a table for crayons or other art materials or moving about the room to choose an object, because this way of moving generates a less self-conscious effort than movement that is more formally orchestrated.

Settling In

As group members arrived, they were given long, narrow pieces of paper folded accordion style, so that there were 10 connected individual pages that folded up into a book. Drawing materials were placed on the table, and group members were invited to represent something about themselves on that day's page. They were then asked to say something about what they created. This could be as simple as "This is just a squiggle," or "I don't know what I am feeling," or it could be something very specific such as "This color green represents the green grass outside," "These are the flowers by the side of my house when I was young; I would feel so happy when they were in bloom," or "This is the deep, dark cloud of depression that is my existence."

Given the 1-hour time frame for the group, this settling in activity needed to be quickly completed within the allotted 5–10 minutes. The emphasis was not on the quality of the representation but on the expression in the moment: "This is me now. This is how I am making meaning now." For some, the pages were related to one another and told a story. For others, they were reflections of internal disjunction. Regardless, each week the marks were inevitably unique. Even if they were similar to those on the previous pages, they had unique degrees of pressure, color, tone, and shape. Similarities representing constancy over time and differences reflecting feeling states that change with time were recognized and underscored in the discussion.

The completed book when folded was the size of a personal safety card often used by domestic violence organizations. The size was small enough to fit into a shoe or pocket and could be carried about without being noticed. These books, once completed at the end of the group, were reminders of constancy, variation, capacity for creative play, and interpersonal connectedness.

This settling-in drawing activity was a form of solitary and parallel play, although the group members were also able to pause and be onlookers. Observing another's process or sharing with another brought them into associative and collaborative cooperative activity. Casual conversation and bonding began to occur around an activity that was not about the trauma. It is important to note that none of the play activities focused on traumatic material but rather reflected more everyday, real-world types of interaction. For example, during an early session one group member mentioned a song she liked and others spontaneously began singing refrains. Barbara found the song on her iPod and played it and everyone sang along. This led to each group member requesting songs for the subsequent weeks and the group establishing a playlist for background music during the weekly settling-in activity.

Topics

We adhered to the topics of the original TIG, incorporating activities, such as mindful movement, playing games, creating art, and even bread-making, that could be related metaphorically to the topics. For example, during the discussion on anger, our activity was bread-making, which entailed working in pairs to read a recipe, mix the ingredients, and knead the dough. Reading a recipe together called for collaboration and communication. The activity was messy and required a physical use of controlled strength for the purpose of strengthening the gluten strands that give the bread its structure. The discussion was about the "messy" communication that can result in destructive expression of anger or in a strengthening of a relationship when approached without the intention to harm or control. Once kneaded, the dough was placed in disposable bread pans to take home, let rise, and then bake.

Approaching this topic, group members had expressed their worries and anxieties about the potential for being emotionally overwhelmed by memories of others' anger or their own. The early collaborative and cooperative aspects of the bread-making activity, coupled with the uniqueness of the activity, distracted members from their fears. It was not long before we were all coated in flour, pulling sticky dough from our fingers and laughing together. In this context, we began to discuss the constructive and destructive potential of anger.

In the next group session, members discussed baking the bread at home with their children and talking about anger with them, and shared fond childhood memories of cooking with grandparents or sad memories of never having home-cooked meals. The associations were both pleasurable and sorrowful, and the group was able to hold them together. The narratives of their lives were gaining texture and shading; they were less black and white than when the group began.

This format was followed each week with a different pairing of activity with topic. For example, we paired the topic "Trust" with creating recipes for trust. The recipes included listing ingredients, such as "a pinch of curiosity and an arm's length of judgment," and the process involved both preparation and cooking, "allowing time for the feelings to rise to the surface before adding the next ingredient." For the group on Relationships, we created yarn bracelets by passing a ball of yarn spontaneously from one group member to another, holding the yarn while passing to create a web of yarn. On each pass, the group member said something about herself to bring her more and more into a "relationship" with the group. The yarn web was then cut into equal parts and turned into bracelets for each group member. For the Body Image topic, we wrote letters to our younger selves, offering compassion, perspective, and validation, and for the Shame topic, we made rag dolls. In this group, having a model on hand and demonstrating how a simple rag doll can be made by tying yarn, twisting pipe cleaners, and wrapping material around stuffing eased any initial doubts that dolls could be so easily created. These dolls are very meaningful for group members, and the discussion that occurred while making the dolls often had elements of both delight and sorrow. Stories of past shame were shared, while members imbued the dolls with a sense of pride and generativity.

There are many activities that could serve these functions, and these are only a few examples. We have also used map making, board game construction, and song writing (rap songs work well). Whichever activity is paired with the topic, it is important to have materials readily on hand and well organized. Instructions should be simple and clear, and the emphasis should be on the process of creating rather than on the end product. Time constraints actually help in this regard, as with only 20–30 minutes per activity, the activities retain spontaneity and playfulness and diminish self-consciousness.

For the closing time of each session, we returned to our chairs to reconnect with ourselves, with one another, and as a group. Each group member had an opportunity to say what she would like to take with her from the session. If there was anything she wanted to leave in the room, she was encouraged to identify that as well.

Closing is essential, as it marks the transition from one space to another. Articulation of the purpose of this time can help group members create a transition for themselves, or at least recognize that the transition is about to occur and that attention to self-regulation skills can be useful.

MALE SURVIVORS GROUP

The VOV Program's male survivor group is another adaptation of the TIG. In this case, the population served was the variable driving the adaptation. Over recent years, as the number of male patients reporting histories of trauma increased, we considered how best to address their needs in a group. Our initial premise, based on a common stereotype, was that men might not be drawn to the same relational model as women. Rather, we thought that men might respond better to a more "businesslike" approach, whereby discussions centered not on feelings, but rather on a topic that would be relevant to most male survivors. For these reasons, the first groups were conducted with a more "educational" focus rather than the relational focus of the TIG. Rather than having two co-leaders seated among the group members, this initial iteration of the group had one co-leader seated with them and the other standing at a whiteboard, writing. This setup gave the group more of a "classroom" feeling rather than relational group energy.

Because this design was experimental, we added an "exit interview" on completion of the group. What came out of those conversations were a number of suggestions for ways to improve the group model. One of the first recommendations was to get rid of the whiteboard and stop using the "classroom" approach, which the men felt had stifled interpersonal bonding. It turned out that the men were as just as hungry as women were for relational connection.

Another recommendation was for the group to aim for an all-male leadership model, which is how the group is currently conducted. At the group's inception, our thinking was that having a female co-leader might help to diminish homophobia in the group. However, over time, the male co-leader began to notice that whenever his female co-leader was absent from the group, the men discussed issues that they did not bring up when she was present. Furthermore, during exit interviews, the group members said that they would feel more comfortable with the group being conducted only by men, not out of any antipathy toward women, but rather because sharing some of their most shaming feelings in the presence of a woman was more painful. The feeling was that the men found it easier to discuss issues that were particularly uncomfortable or embarrassing for them, like sexual dysfunction, only with other men, because the presence of a female co-leader heightened their self-consciousness, shame, and humiliation and made their feelings too hard to bear. (It is important to note that the Boston Area Rape Crisis Center, which serves a different population from our mental health clinic, has successfully adapted the TIG model for male survivors with male and female co-leaders.)

Another recommendation by the members was that the number and length of group sessions be extended to allow for more discussion. Over the years, the group has evolved from a 60-minute group for 10 weeks, to a 75-minute group for 12 weeks, to a 90-minute group for 16 weeks, which is the current iteration of the model. This extension in time and duration has allowed the group to offer its members more opportunity to discuss the ways in which their traumatic pasts influence their lives today. It has promoted a deeper connection among the men, and their relational capacity has served as a powerful antidote to their social isolation and self-blame. As part of this evolution, the group has become what the VOV Program now refers to as a "hybridized model," meaning simply that it has progressed somewhat beyond the classic Stage 1 group, focusing purely on psychoeducation, safety, and self-care, and has taken on some features of a Stage 2 model, focused on a trauma narrative. More precisely, the group could be described as a "Stage 1½." It allows time for more sharing and discussion, but members are still advised against telling their stories in the kind of depth and detail that occurs in a classic Stage 2 group.

Another adaptation for the male survivor group involves the screening process. During an initial phone interview, prospective patients are asked standard questions that would rule out inclusion in the group. In addition to standard questions about active substance abuse, psychosis, suicidal ideation, recent hospitalization, and unstable or dangerous living situations, male patients are asked about active perpetration. We include this question based on the fact that male survivors of childhood abuse are at increased risk of perpetrating sexual and domestic violence. Some survivors may have perpetrated such violence as children or adolescents, possibly under duress. As long as the survivor expresses remorse for this behavior and makes it clear that it is no longer occurring, it is not grounds for exclusion. In fact, it can be an important part of group sharing by helping group members address the common fear that male survivors are doomed to become perpetrators (in fact, the great majority do not).

If after the brief phone screening the group leader and the prospective patient think that this group may be a good fit, the patient is invited for an in-person interview. During this interview, the patient is asked many questions about his traumatic past and the ways in which it continues to influence his life today. Part of the motivation behind this line of inquiry is to check for the patient's ability to reference traumatic material without becoming triggered or overwhelmed. The patient is informed that although no explicit details of his traumatic past will be shared in this group, one of the goals of the group is to help men identify their experience and receive validation and support for what they have survived. For example, one patient explained in his interview that he was a survivor of incest perpetrated by his father when he was a teenager. He felt that this traumatic experience left him unable to have intimate relationships because of strong feelings of shame and guilt. The group leader encouraged this man to share his story in the group, but without giving any details of the actual acts of incest.

Because this group can be so emotionally stirring, in spite of its highly structured nature, during the course of the group each man is asked to name a person to whom he can turn for additional support. Often, the man will cite his individual therapist, but for those men who are not currently in treatment, the group leader explores other resources whom they can seek out. Frequently, the patient may return to a previous therapist for a period of time-limited work, or he may see his AA sponsor more frequently or increase the number of AA or NA groups he attends. Early on, the group had an expectation that each member would have a current individual therapist but, over time, the group leaders realized that having one was not really necessary for all survivors. Some men who had years of individual treatment prior to their joining the group did not feel the need to continue in individual therapy. In fact, they preferred to have the support of an entire group of male survivors.

If a man is currently in therapy, he is asked to sign a consent form for the group leaders to confer with his therapist. After securing consent, one of the group leaders will call the client's therapist to discuss the therapist's sense of the patient's readiness for group and any concerns the therapist may have. The group leader will also ask the therapist for ideas about possible goals for the patient to work on in this group.

Another important part of the screening process is to address a particular issue relevant to an all-male population—the problem of homophobia. The group leaders speak with each man about his feelings about being in a group with men of diverse sexual orientations. Each member is told that there may be men in the group who identify as gay, straight, bisexual, or transgender. He is then asked how he feels about being in a group with these men. If the man responds by saying that he feels discomfort at this prospect, then he would be asked to consider another group in lieu of this one.

The group leaders try to avoid having any member become tokenized, meaning that they try to prevent there being only one openly straight or one openly gay man, for example, in each group. Historically, in terms of race and ethnicity, the group has been predominantly, but not exclusively, white, composed of men with a Western European heritage. There has been much more diversity around age, with members ranging from a youthful 19 to a mature 74 years.

During the screening for the male survivor group, each man was asked to identify at least one goal that he would like to accomplish during the group, and his initial aspirations were recorded verbatim. Their statements made it clear that issues of identity and relationship were their central concerns. Some examples from recent groups include:

"I want to feel like I am part of the human race."

"I don't want to have to act macho all the time, when I actually feel scared much of the time."

"I would like to learn how to make a friend."

"I want to feel less alone and feel less bad about myself."

"I wish that I didn't have to feel so defective."

"I want to stop believing that I caused the sexual abuse because I am gay."

"I don't want to hate myself anymore."

"I want to try to be a better father."

"I want to learn who I am, and I want to stop believing that I am that person that my abuser convinced me that I was."

"I have to learn how to stop being such an asshole."

Goal setting is not a standard feature of the TIG. The inclusion of a goal is an adaptation from our Stage 2 group model. Because many men generate goals that could not possibly be accomplished during a time-limited group, the group leaders collaborate with each member to concretize a more measurable and achievable goal. Some of those goals have included disclosing to a partner that he is participating in this group; attending each and every group session; participating verbally in every group by sharing at least one reaction to the material; making eye contact with other members during every group session; bringing one's reaction to each group back to one's individual therapist for further exploration; and adding in a new self-care routine for the duration of the group.

Other common goals men have identified over the years are "I want to be able to sit in a room with other men and say that I'm a survivor of sexual abuse that was done against me when I was only a boy" or "I want to hear how other men cope with the trauma and how it comes up now so I can learn to cope." Another example, which was articulated quite poignantly by a recent group member, was, "I want to be able to ask other men who were sexually abused as kids how they answer the question 'How old were you when you lost your virginity?' How do I answer that question? I get asked that all the time by friends and guys at work, and I never know what to say. Do I say, 'When I was 7 and abused by my older brother,' or do I say, 'When I was 20 and had my first real girlfriend?'"

Typically, in the first couple of weeks of the group, the men share the goals they hope to accomplish. Because this goal formation was discussed with the group leaders during the initial screening, and the group leaders helped to shape concrete goals that could be easily accomplished during the course of the group, the members openly comment when they notice that a member is explicitly working on a goal. From the preceding examples, the group may cheer a man on when he candidly discusses his realization that he gets to decide when he had his first sexual experience, and that it doesn't have to have anything to do with the first time he was sexually abused. In fact, the group will help him recognize that being sexually abused was an act of violence, not of sex, and therefore the first time he engaged in sex consensually was when he "lost his virginity." The tracking of each man's goal does not usually take up a significant portion of group time, but it is openly stated and noted throughout the group sessions. In the final session, when members are discussing their experience in the group, goal completion is often paramount in contributing to what made the group feel successful to them.

Other than the addition of the goal, the male survivor group follows the basic structure of the TIG. It opens with a settling in, which sometimes includes deep breathing or a relaxation exercise, but often occurs in silence. One can see the growing comfort they have with one another as the weeks pass. The group always begins with an opening check-in, during which we hear how the men are feeling as they arrive in the group and if there is anything from the previous week that has stayed with them or troubled them that they would like to review. The group then moves into what we call the working part of the group, in which the members read the week's handout and discuss the impact that their traumatic past has on their lives today within the context of whatever topic we happen to be discussing that particular week. Finally, the group ends with a closing round, which is a final check-in where each member reports how he is feeling as he departs the group. As part of this phase, he also names one self-care task he can engage in before the next week's group. Most topics are discussed within 1 week, but sometimes we take 2 weeks to explore a topic. We always save discussion of the more evocative topics for later sessions to allow time for greater group cohesion and bonding to develop among the members.

Sometimes a specific topic will result in homework for a member. For example, in a 2-week session on anger, the group asked one member to go home and take notes on what was happening in his relationship with his wife that resulted in a chronic sense of anger toward her because he didn't seem to have any data to explain his anger, to the group or even to himself. The man returned the following week and read a few journal entries to the group. As he did so, he began to gain insight into how reactive he became when he interpreted his wife's most innocuous comments as critical and disapproving. He was then able to notice how his wife often reminded him of the critical and verbally abusive mother of his childhood. With this insight, he was able to step back from his anger.

As illustrated in the following brief vignette, some men take real risks. In the first week of a 2-week session on sex and sexuality, one group member with the pseudonym Sean revealed something very painful just at the very end of the topic discussion: "I am ashamed to admit this," he said, "but during the years of sexual abuse by my cousin, I went back to him repeatedly, even after I should have been old enough to make him stop, but I wanted to go back." Unfortunately, this brave disclosure fell flat with the other members. No one responded, and all the men sat in silence. Sean looked shamed by the group's silence. He sat with his head bowed, his shoulders slumped, and his eyes fixed on a spot on the floor. The group leaders tried unsuccessfully both to acknowledge Sean's courage and to engage the group. When it came time for the closing round, Sean passed. The group leaders asked to check in with him after the group session, but he reassured them that he was fine; he just wanted to go home.

The following week, Sam, one of the other group members, spoke up. He said to Sean, "I am so sorry that I didn't respond to you last week when you revealed what you did with your cousin. The reason I didn't is because I did the exact same thing. I, too, used to go back to my perpetrator for sex, even though I knew it was wrong. I just didn't have the courage to tell you that last week."

Justin, another member, concurred, saying, "For me, I feel guilty, too, that I didn't respond to you last week. As I mentioned in earlier groups, my father sexually abused me. However, what I didn't share with you was that although the abuse began when I now know I was too small to stop it, it continued past the time I could have made him stop. The truth is that I let it continue because it was only at night, in those few minutes when my father would come into my room, that I ever felt close to him, and in some way even loved. I sure didn't feel it during the day or any other time. I realize now that desiring his love and approval made me hate myself more and more."

What is striking in this vignette is that in the previous week, the men had done what could be refered to as "the locker-room thing." Someone had brought up having an issue with pornography and masturbation, and there was a lot of laughter among the guys, in a "towel-snapping" kind of way. When Sean revealed what he did about returning to his perpetrator, his disclosure fell flat. But by the following week, the men were able to move to a place of real honesty, compassion, and empathy. They were able to establish a genuine connection by having the courage to allow themselves to be vulnerable in such an authentic way. It was a very powerful moment to witness.

During a session on the topic Relationships, one member said, "You know what I realize I am missing in my life? A real friend. I used to see two guys having dinner together, or going to the movies together, and I would assume that they must be gay. You know, I haven't had a real friend since I was a boy, and I recognize now that is what I am longing for, that in some ways, that is what I miss most." The other members of the group engaged in a conversation about the meaning of friendship and how for some of them, it had been too frightening to even entertain the idea of a male friend because they were so burdened by homophobia.

In a session focused on recovery and healing, a man named Paul said, "I have a son and a daughter, and I am not close to them at all; it is like there is this invisible wall between us, and I don't know how to cross it." The group responded by encouraging him to try to find ways to engage with them more and to try to get to know them better. Paul said, "You know, I don't believe that my children have ever been abused because they are great kids and not screwed up at all like I was at their age. I can thank my ex-wife for that. If I could have anything in the world, I would want to be close to them because I can see that they want that too. I used to be too afraid to get close because I had this feeling that what is wrong with me would somehow rub off on them, like they would become contaminated by the poison I have always felt is inside of me. Sometimes I cannot believe the price I have paid for what was done to me."

Another group member, Terence, described knowing from the time he was a child that he was gay, or "queer," the descriptor used when he was a child, and also knowing how homophobic his family was. So when a group of senior boys cornered him and gang-raped him when he was a freshman, he didn't tell anyone for fear of being "outed." One of the most painful aspects of being raped was not only the physical pain he suffered, but also the shame and humiliation he felt because of the degrading names his attackers called him. For months after the assault, the attackers whispered these names when they passed him in the hall or in the bathrooms. They were especially wounding because they were the same words that his father used at home. He recalled how his father would often tell him, "I would never be a man." Terence went on to share the difficulty he has always found in all-male environments, and how challenging it was to consider joining the male survivor group in spite of his therapist's urging to do so over the years.

Another group member, Max, responded to Terence, saying that he found him to be a man based on the way Terence responded so respectfully and compassionately to the other group members. In addition, Max said that he felt that Terence was a wonderful example of a courageous man, one who took the risk to join an all-male group despite his reservations and personal history. He noted how courageous he must have been as an adolescent to survive in the toxic atmosphere of the school and at home with his family. Terence became visibly moved by this feedback. He said that no other man had ever told him he had courage before, and it so contrasted with his own self-concept of being a "coward." The group leader added that perhaps Terence could begin to replace some of the self-denigrating names he has been burdened with all these years with new descriptors, like courageous and compassionate. In addition, the group leader said that at the VOV Program, many survivors have talked about how it is easier to recover from physical and sexual abuse than it is from verbal abuse because verbal abuse is so insidious and seems to be carried on almost a cellular level. Terence cried for just a few moments and then said that he was grateful to be in a room of men who seemed so invested in healing and in recovering rather than in hurting others as a way to make themselves feel better.

Although the session is always focused on the topic of recovery and the next steps, for the final week of the group sometimes instead of a worksheet, the men may be given a structured exercise. The following guideline has proved popular.

> "Using 3-2-1, please think of *three* things you got from group that you consider valuable; *two* supports you have in the world; and *one* next step for yourself in your journey of recovery."

After the group ends each man is invited back for an exit interview. During this conversation, he is asked to share what he found useful in the group in terms of the group structure and content of the handouts, as well as what he wishes had been different about the group. He is told that his feedback has real value, and that the group leaders owe a debt to group members who came before him, as they have helped to shape the group into the form it currently has. In addition to asking the men for group feedback, the group leaders give specific suggestions to each member regarding their recommendations for his next steps. For example, the group leaders may suggest that the member attend another trauma group, or that he consider a different treatment modality, or that he do specific time-limited work in individual therapy. As at the start of group, if the patient has an individual therapist, the group leaders confer with the therapist and pass along their treatment recommendations.

In the final meeting of the group, and in exit interviews, men have summed up their experience in these words:

> "I don't have any illusion that I am all healed now, but at least I have more hope."
> "I used to feel like a freak, but at least now I feel more human."

"Even though I still don't have any real friends, I now feel like I might actually make one at some point."

"The most important thing I got out of this group is that I don't feel so alone, or like I caused the abuse."

"I feel like I can salvage at least the remainder of my life if I get to work on this stuff."

"Even though I was made to have sex all those years, my abuser didn't take away my manhood, like I always thought he did."

"I spent the first 40 years of my life believing that the abuse was my fault, and now I finally believe that it wasn't."

"I deserve more in life than I have, and I am going to try to get it."

MI JARDÍN INTERIOR: A GROUP FOR LATINA IMMIGRANTS

This adaptation of the TIG model was developed by Rosa Maria Bramble, a licensed clinical social worker in New York. Ms. Bramble is a participant in a monthly conference call, co-led by Judith Herman and Emily Schatzow, MEd, in which they consult on group therapy for trauma survivors. Here, what drives the adaptation is the need to make the TIG model culturally acceptable to the Latina immigrant population and to make the content of the sessions more relevant to the kinds of traumas that these women most commonly endure. "The beauty of the model," says Bramble, "is that it allows for introducing the idea of trauma in our culture" (personal communication with J. L. Herman, November 7, 2016).

Bramble notes that Latina immigrants are at a high risk for many forms of trauma, first in their country of origin where they may be exposed to political or gang violence, as well as domestic violence and child abuse. Many women flee violence by crossing the borders and risk their lives in the process. During migration, they are often exposed to further violence in the form of sexual assault, kidnapping, and human trafficking, and finally, they may face multiple stressors once they arrive in the United States since they are often undocumented. Undocumented women are also more vulnerable if they become involved in abusive relationships postmigration because the abuser can use threats of deportation as a form of control. Despite higher rates of trauma, PTSD, and depression, Latina immigrants are less likely than women in other ethnic groups to seek mental health care. Shame associated with migration trauma or undocumented status, cultural stigma against mental illness, and a fear of being perceived as *loca* (crazy) are barriers to treatment. As Bramble points out, Latino culture also values resilience and believes that people should be able to handle their own affairs.

Bramble writes:

My clinical experience supports the concept of belongingness with other "compañeras" (compatriots) . . . as together they share stories of challenges and resilience. Therefore, a group model, such as the TIG, may be the most effective in addressing the multiple needs of immigrant Latinas with trauma and PTSD. TIG adaptation to Latinas is culturally informed and integrates the realities of immigration status and the sociopolitical realities of Latinas. (personal communication with J. L. Herman, November 7, 2016)

Bramble offers the following adaptation guidelines:

1. The name "TIG" makes people anxious and turns them off. We changed it to "My Inner Garden: Strengthening My Emotional Health," a name that offers a vision of resilience. The flyer clarifies that the group is for trauma survivors.
2. For Latinas, we need to acknowledge the level of literacy, and we provide options. We do not go around the room [reading from worksheets], but rather let participants volunteer to read.
3. Latinas are a heterogeneous group. As part of creating safety in the group, we recognize that participants come from different countries, and we embrace and welcome all. This is a good transition to the discussion of how we are all affected by trauma.
4. We spend time distinguishing trauma from depression—trauma is new! Latinas will more readily say "I'm depressed," rather than "I was traumatized." There is a lack of precise language to explain and understand trauma.
5. In our adaptation for Latinas, we realized it was important to include the following additional core topics and worksheets:
   • Trauma of migration.
   • Impact of trauma on children and families.
   • Trauma of discrimination and undocumented status.
6. Zumba, a type of music popular with Latinas, is used to connect to a positive self-image within a cultural context. Group members learned to regulate their breathing while moving to the rhythms.
7. Finally, the last group session is devoted to a celebration, in which food as well as music is shared.

Bramble also varied the length of the groups. She developed two different variations for two different agencies: one group lasting 6 weeks and the other 9 weeks. Groups were offered in the evenings or on Saturdays so that clients would not miss employment opportunities. The groups were conducted in Spanish, with Spanish translations of the worksheets (provided in an online supplement to this book; see box at end of Table of Contents for details).

In *Mi Jardín Interior*, adaptations were made in all three ecological variables: the population, parameters, and environmental setting of the group. Nevertheless, the basic structures or "bones" of the group were maintained.

THE TRAUMA INFORMATION
GROUP OBSERVATION MODEL

For those who feel an affinity for this group model, who have become well versed in its approach, and who have a well-integrated understanding of both trauma theory and group processes, pairing an observed group with the manual can provide a rich learning experience for both group participants and observers alike.

At the VOV Program, Lois Glass has adapted the group for training of clinicians and allied health providers. In this observed group model, group members are not only beginning to organize their own experiences into meaningful frameworks of compassionate understanding and enhancing the well-being of their fellow group members, but they are also broadening and enriching the trauma sensitivity of providers. They become change agents.

How it Works

In this observed training model, the TIG is conducted as it is described in this manual, but there are important changes to the screening process and to the first and last group sessions. Additionally, the leaders facilitate an hour of discussion for the observers each week after the group.

Screening

The screening phone call is oriented around the information that this group will be observed, the rationale for doing so, and the practical details about the observation process. For example, the group leader might say, "We believe that it is important to teach others how to work with trauma survivors, and one very helpful way is to teach through observation, followed by an opportunity for discussion." Practically group observation occurs by means of a video camera or a "one-way mirror" on one wall of the room through which the group meeting can be seen from the adjacent room, where observers will be sitting. The observers are the clinicians and allied health professionals who want to learn more about how traumatic events impact people and how to be sensitive to this impact in their interactions. The observers attend every week, and they need to abide by the same rules of confidentiality that we ask the members of the group to maintain. For example, were any of the observers acquainted with any of the group members, they would be asked to excuse themselves immediately to ensure that members do not have to worry about being observed by a neighbor or acquaintance.

The group leaders also explain that for a few minutes at the end of the first session the observers will be invited into the group to introduce themselves and that they will be invited in again at the end of the last session to give feedback. Group members will have the option to stay and meet the observers or to leave before they come in.

The rationale for the initial introduction is to establish transparency and to reduce the feeling of the unknown or of voyeurism. The meeting also seals an implicit contract of respect and confidentiality between the two groups. (Group members also sign an explicit consent form for the observation during the initial screening meeting.) With these contracts in place, group members can focus on the work at hand: their process of recovery. Lois reports that after the first week or so, members report only a visceral sense of others in the adjacent room, which may be heightened briefly if an observer comes in late, causing a light to flicker across the mirror. At other times a member may speak directly to the observers, either to make a point or when shame threatens to overcome her. The skillful group leader addresses this issue directly by including the observers' role of witnesses in the group process of recovery from shame.

The Observers' Group

The first observers' group starts with an explanation about the observed group model, which follows the flow of the manual. Each aspect of the group model is reviewed. This leads into brief introductions of each observer. Any remaining time left is set aside for observers' questions.

All subsequent discussion sessions begin with questions and issues raised by the observers and then segues into teaching moments chosen by the leader(s). Discussion is also tailored to the specific profession and work environment of the observer. For example, if there were an addictions counselor among the observers, the leader would highlight the interplay between addictions and trauma. There might also be a discussion about whether to recommend a survivors' group for a patient in individual therapy and how to explain this group model in language most likely to resonate with the patient's experience.

Observers are often interested in the therapists' interventions. This provides an opportunity for the group leaders to talk about their thinking process while conducting the group and how they chose the interventions they used. Nuanced discussion often follows, affording another opportunity for the group leaders to be transparent about their countertransference and/or vicarious traumatization. One of the most useful aspects of the observation group is illuminating the process of untangling a complex group interaction. Hearing a group leader say, "Had I had more perspective, or more time to reflect, I might have said . . . , but there was so much going on . . . and sometimes a group leader can't attend to everything" can be very reassuring, especially when the statement is followed by showing how to recover these "lost opportunities" when coming back to the topic the following week. Normalization, clarification, and validation are as essential to the supervisory relationship as they are to the therapeutic one.

Week 10: The Final Group Session

At the end of this final group session, the observers are invited back to meet with the group members once again. Those group members who prefer to leave prior to this meeting may do so. Without exception, these meetings underscore the transformative power of active listening and active witnessing. Each observer has an opportunity to say what he or she has learned from the group members and the group process. The feedback honors the suffering that the group members so courageously allowed themselves to reveal and the compassionate way they offered solace to others. Each group member's participation brings into vivid and heartfelt relief how the pathways of recovery are both similar and unique. Common to all is that the journey along these pathways is eased when aided by trauma-informed knowledge, compassion, and respect.

CONCLUSION

The risk of manualizing any group model is that the manual is interpreted and followed so literally that the manual overrides real-world experience. As you can see from the examples of these TIG adaptations, we hope that this manual offers a structural framework from which effective adaptations may arise.

We think of the group model as a living organism, dynamic in its interplay between purpose, structure, theory of change, the participants' traumas, and the cultural context of their lives. We have also identified group models as serving the function of a "home base" and "safe place" for group members and likened their essential elements to the "bones and bearing walls" that support the integrity of the group structure. These are the key theoretical constructs that need to be preserved when adapting the group model.

We can see how the concept of safety, an essential aspect of the theory of recovery from trauma, is a fundamental theoretical underpinning of all the adaptations, while each group has been tailored to fit the population served and, to some extent, the personality of the group leaders. In the group *Mi Jardín Interior*, the name of the group was changed to offset the anxiety associated with the direct naming of trauma, the topics were adapted to suit the experience of this population, and music and food were introduced to offer cultural resonance. This attention to culture, language, and the experience of trauma influenced the design of the group, while promoting safe participation. In the Passageways group, play activities and natural movement, through displacement, helped members connect with their resilient capabilities prior to the discussion of the impact of trauma. In the Male Survivors Group, safety was enhanced by seeking feedback that resulted in adapting the leadership to be more sensitive to the potential for shame. Group members were also asked to identify supports in their environment to decrease isolation.

In each of the adaptations described in this chapter, the three structural elements of a beginning (opening exercise), middle (topics and discussion), and ending (closing round) have been maintained. Variation occurs in the topical content of each of these elements and in the therapeutic approach, which may incorporate meditation, art therapy, music, or dance techniques. Variation may also occur in practical matters, such as the length or number of sessions or the number of group members. The philosophical and theoretical underpinnings, however, remain the same.

A fourth element described more fully in the earlier chapters and in the description of the male survivor group is the screening process. How group leaders screen is determined by many factors—all of which must align with the purpose of the group, comfort level of the group leaders, and amount of traumatic material being explored. For example, the TIG incorporating play and creative activities group screens only by phone. The purpose of the screening is to inform the prospective group member about the format of the group and what to expect. It clarifies misunderstandings and unrealistic expectations. Only after these initial matters are discussed does the group leader begin to gather information about the prospective group member. Information gathered is limited to current functioning, interests, life circumstances, and a very general history. No traumatic details are brought up because they are not discussed in the group. This sets the tone for the group participation.

Inquiring about interests aligns with the emphasis on creative and playful activities and building resiliency skills that is a focus of this group. The male survivors group, on the other hand, has a more in-depth trauma screening since that group is designed to allow for the processing of traumatic material. This design includes an extended time frame (in both the length of each session and the duration of the group) and goal setting, which provides a structure and purpose for discussing the current life impact of traumatic events.

All of the group adaptations use core topics as an organizing framework, but each approaches the topics uniquely. The Passageways group follows the sequencing of the topics of the TIG, but doesn't introduce the worksheets into the discussion. The worksheets are seen as resources and are handed out for home use or to be used during individual therapy. *Mi Jardín Interior,* which is sensitive to literacy levels, group members volunteer to read from the worksheets, and the topics are adapted to suit the language and cultural experience of the group members. The male survivors group began as more of a classroom model, with the leaders standing in front of the group at a whiteboard reviewing the worksheets, then evolved to a more interactive and collaborative group process, in which the leaders and members read the worksheets together and then begin a discussion and homework assigned through a collaborative process with the group leader. Adaptations in group models occur "in the moment," as well as in the planning stages.

Another variable we recognize is the individuality of the group leaders. In each of the adaptations described, perhaps you can feel the personality of the group leaders shining through. It is important that group leaders be authentic, that their voices be clear, ring true, and resonate with a thorough understanding of the material, and that they be knowledgeable about trauma and the principles of recovery and comfortable with the group process.

In summary, the questions that guide our adaptations are "Why this adaptation?"; "Am I maintaining the 'bones and bearing walls' that support this model?"; "Am I comfortable in my role?"; "Where am I going and why?" Once we have the answers, the adaptation process begins.

We return to Alice, but unlike her, we set our course prior to setting forth.

> "—so long as I get SOMEWHERE," Alice added as an explanation.
> "Oh, you're sure to do that," said the Cat, "if you only walk long enough."
> —Lewis Carroll, *Alice's Adventures in Wonderland* (2011)

Schedule for the Trauma Information Group

This group consists of 10 self-contained, topic-oriented sessions, with the goal of providing the members with a greater understanding of trauma, the psychological aftermath of victimization, and the process of recovery. The emphasis will be on providing a framework for understanding trauma so that members can achieve some mastery of their therapeutic work. We will utilize worksheets and handouts, which members may later bring to their individual therapy for further exploration and individual processing.

The group will meet on _____ from _____ to _____.

Session 1	The Impact of Trauma: Posttraumatic Stress Reactions
Session 2	Safety and Self-Care
Session 3	Trust
Session 4	Remembering
Session 5	Shame and Self-Blame
Session 6	Compassion
Session 7	Anger
Session 8	Self-Image/Body Image
Session 9	Relationships with and Connections to Others
Session 10	Meaning Making of the Past and the Process of Recovery

Guidelines for the Trauma Information Group

1. Group members are encouraged to attend every group. If you are unable to attend a group, please let us know in advance so other members will not worry. You can leave a message for us at _____.

2. There is no food allowed in the group. Food can be a distraction, as well as a sensitive issue for other group members. Water and nonalcoholic drinks are okay.

3. It is very important to maintain confidentiality in the group. We want you to talk in general terms about the group with family and friends. Care should be taken not to refer to anyone by name.

4. If you know or encounter group members outside of the group, we ask that you not discuss either the group or your trauma histories.

5. In order to maintain membership in the group, individuals need to be in safe living situations, be able to commit to a safety plan, and be able to maintain sobriety. If you are struggling with these issues, we will check with you to evaluate the advisability of remaining in the group.

6. This group focuses on the ways in which traumatic experiences have impacted and continue to impact your lives, how you cope with these effects, and your progress in recovering from them. Our goal is to help people develop a cognitive framework for understanding their experience in a setting that offers support and challenges feelings of isolation. The content and specifics of people's trauma histories will not be a focus of the group. In addition, this is not a group that focuses on the reactions of members to each other. We ask that you bring these issues to individual therapy or to your other supports.

APPENDIX C
Trauma Information Group Handouts and Worksheets

Session 1. The Impact of Trauma: Posttraumatic Stress Reactions

What Is a Traumatic Event?

Traumatic events are events that cause or threaten to cause physical, emotional, and psychological harm. They include rape, child abuse, battering, and other threats to one's life and/or physical or emotional integrity. They may also include natural disasters, accidents, domestic terrorism, or wartime experiences, which are not the focus of this group.

Traumatic events overwhelm a person's coping capacities and result in feeling out of control and experiencing intense fear and helplessness. Traumatic events are often experienced by survivors as incomprehensible and senseless.

What Are Typical (Understandable, Expected) Reactions?

People respond to traumatic experiences in a variety of ways. Different people may respond differently to the same traumatic event. Some will have immediate responses, while others will have responses that are delayed. Delayed responses can occur even years after the original event because people may "run out of steam" for their initial ways of coping, such as avoidance, hard work, or alcohol or substance abuse, or they may be stopped in their tracks by some new loss or even a physical injury. At such times, they can feel that the impact of trauma "catches up" with them.

An individual does not have to experience the trauma directly to be affected. Eyewitnesses, loved ones, and caregivers can be affected as a result of having seen or heard about frightening and/or incomprehensible violence.

Although each person reacts differently according to his or her personality, past experiences, connection to the event, the response of others, and the meaning given to the event, there are common feelings and reactions that frequently occur after a person has been involved in or witnessed a traumatic or violent event(s).

How Do People Respond to Traumatic Events?

Experiencing trauma can affect almost every aspect of one's life: how one thinks, feels emotionally and physically, acts, and relates to others, as well as one's spiritual faith or beliefs about the world and people. The following table is a list of common reactions. Any combination of these or similar reactions can be considered a "normal" response to a traumatic event or series of events.

(continued)

How One Thinks	**How One Acts**	**One's Beliefs or Spirituality**
difficulty remembering difficulty making decisions confusion time distortion too many thoughts at once slowed-down thinking feeling that the world is not safe thinking about dying flashbacks—reexperiencing the event intrusive images—replaying the event sense of foreshortened future	abusing drugs, alcohol, medication withdrawing from others impatience irritability easily "swamped" strong reactions to small changes clinging to people inability to perform skills once easily accomplished disruption of daily routine	loss of faith spiritual doubts withdrawal from religious community questioning old beliefs sense of the world being changed despair life feels meaningless
How One Feels Emotionally	**How One Feels Physically**	**How One Relates to Others**
helpless, hopeless, powerless grief numbness dread/fear/safety concerns guilt feeling vulnerable/dependent anger/rage emotional roller coaster nightmares feeling worthless feeling alone feeling a lack of a sense of control over one's life feeling of uncleanness fear of what other people might think fear of ongoing victimization	fatigue changes in sleep eating/appetite problems stomach problems vomiting/diarrhea sweating/rapid pulse chest pains dizziness/headaches easily catch colds/feel sick back/neck pain	difficulty trusting people at all trusting too much, too soon changes in sexual activity distorted generalizations about others doubts about relationships choosing partners who turn out to be controlling or abusive or reenact trauma dynamics feeling critical of others alienation from family/friends who don't understand sense of aloneness/feeling "not human" fear of ongoing victimization

How Do People Recover from Trauma?

Recovery from trauma is a complicated process that takes time. Throughout this group, we will be exploring different aspects of recovery. As you go through this group, remember that there may be times when you feel more in control of your emotions and times when you might feel more out of control. It is important to take good care of yourself and to recognize that recovery is hard work. Paying attention to your physical, spiritual, and emotional needs can help you feel more in control of your life and reduce the stress involved in recovery. Listed below are basic aspects of daily life to which we encourage you to pay attention. After each one, space is provided for you to write down your strategies for self-care.

(continued)

Diet

In the aftermath of stressful situations people often eat more sugar and drink caffeine to give them a boost. Though these ways of coping initially seem to provide energy, they actually increase overall stress levels. Alcohol and drug use may numb some feelings at the time of use, but they too make feelings worse with time. Think about your diet and how it might be affecting your stress level.

_____

_____

_____

_____

_____

Physical Activity

One of the best ways to reduce stress is to exercise. Exercise is not just fun, it is a very effective way to cope with stress and anxious feelings. Think about your daily routine and how you can begin to include some regular exercise into it.

_____

_____

_____

_____

_____

Rest and Relaxation

Learning to find ways to calm yourself down and to be restful and quiet are other options for counteracting stress. Deep breathing exercises, some forms of meditation, and quiet walks are ways that many people soothe themselves. How do you quiet yourself down?

_____

_____

_____

_____

_____

(continued)

Social Contacts and Support Systems

One of the effects of trauma is that it often leads to isolation. Sometimes people keep to themselves because they are afraid that expressing strong or painful feelings will drive others away. Whatever the reason, isolation usually intensifies these feelings. Finding other people to talk to who can listen to how you feel, and who understand something about what you have been through, can be very helpful. Who can you talk to about how you feel?

_____

_____

_____

_____

_____

_____

Session 2. Safety and Self-Care

For many people who have had traumatic experiences, finding ways to keep themselves safe and taking better care of themselves are the first steps in recovery. In this worksheet, we discuss the ways in which trauma impacts an individual's feeling of safety in the world and how trauma can hinder self-care. Our goal is to focus on how trauma survivors can develop a sense of safety and learn new ways to care for themselves.

Safety

Feeling safe in our world is a complicated task. There are ways in which the world is really not a safe place, and of course, some people and places are safer than others. However, in spite of the uncertainties that surround us, we all need to go through our daily lives without living in fear of immediate danger or bodily harm.

Safety is the experience of feeling cared for and protected from harm. Young children are most likely to develop a sense of safety when the people in the world around them are attentive to their needs, comfort them when they are frightened, and teach them about the many ways to protect themselves. If this nurturing occurs early in life, children have a greater chance of growing into adults who know how to ask for help, how to avoid dangerous situations, and how to judge whether other people are trustworthy. We would say that these people have a basic sense of security in the world.

Traumatic experiences have a profound impact upon our sense of safety. This is true both for survivors who were traumatized as young children and for those who were traumatized as adults. For survivors who were traumatized as children, trust issues are often central in adulthood. This certainly makes sense—if young children are unable to trust those people who should have protected and nurtured them, but were instead repeatedly exposed to harm, they learn that people are not trustworthy. Unprotected children also learn that their safety is not important—that they don't matter enough to be cared for.

If the adults in a child's life were unpredictable—sometimes loving and sometimes hurtful or neglectful—the child may become confused. In such a "hot-and-cold" emotional setting, feelings of safety, fearfulness, aloneness, and panic may have become mixed together. As this child grows up, the words *safety* or *trust* may not make any sense to her. For her, all relationships may revive the confusing and painful mixture of feelings she experienced earlier in her life.

Some survivors learn to protect themselves from painful feelings by "numbing out" or "dissociating." When these survival patterns continue into adulthood, the survivor remains in a state of disconnection. She may feel empty inside or incomplete. Some kinds of feelings—anger, for example—may be completely unavailable, even when they would be appropriate. Life does not seem to make sense.

Other survivors may protect themselves from painful feelings by seeking out ways to alter their awareness through alcohol, drugs, risky sexual encounters, or other forms of self-harm. These ways of coping may make survivors feel more in control of what happens to them. They might seek out harm as self-punishment. They might end promising new relationships, assuming they will be hurt in the end, so they take control of *when* to end them. Or they may use childhood coping skills of "numbing out" or not thinking about danger when they should. In all these ways, the means of self-protection developed in childhood may make survivors less safe in the present.

(continued)

For survivors who were traumatized as adults, safety and self-care issues can also be prominent. Many rape survivors describe limiting their contacts with the outside world in an effort to feel safer and, as a result, may lead very restricted lives. Women who have been battered may close themselves off from others in fear or shame, feeling that being isolated is safest. But people do not heal in isolation. It is vitally important to have a social world. The challenge is how to find safe ways to do it.

Establishing safety means creating a way of life that minimizes your risk of harming yourself or of being harmed by others.

A few of the ways a survivor may compromise her safety include:

- Living in unsafe housing
- Abusing drugs and alcohol
- Entering into abusive relationships
- Not going to the doctor when necessary
- Spending too much money

Self-Care

When a child's sense of self has been violated and her trust betrayed, she learns to hide her feelings and to deny what she needs. She may also feel she does not deserve to care for herself. This behavior can continue into adulthood. She may wear only a sweater in the cold of winter. She may eat only when she is alone, forget to eat altogether, or perhaps eat only junk food. She may sleep only 3 hours a night or perhaps 14. She may live with someone who is abusive to her, or get an apartment where she can't afford to pay the rent. In all of these situations, she is not safe emotionally or physically.

To many survivors, the concept of self-care is as foreign as the concept of safety. Self-care means paying attention to your basic needs and respecting those needs as important and as your right. Self-care starts with your body. It means establishing a structure in your life, with predictable rhythms of sleeping, eating, and activity. It means going to the doctor for medical problems and engaging in therapy, maintaining sobriety if substance abuse has been a problem, and practicing safe sex if you are sexually active. Self-care also extends to your immediate environment and current relationships. It means being able to provide for your basic survival needs. It means making sure that your current living situation is safe and that in your current relationships you are free from intimidation or exploitation.

Practicing self-care builds self-respect and self-confidence. As you begin to feel that you have a right to care, it will become easier to develop new relationships based on mutual support and respect. Learning to use social supports and to reach out to others is another part of the recovery process that can begin once you are practicing good self-care.

Sometimes, despite your best efforts, it can be hard to think of ways to take care of yourself. At these times your emotional pain may be so great that resorting to drugs, drinking, hurting yourself, or withdrawing from others may seem to be the only options you have. But they bring relief only in the short run, while in the long run they isolate you even more. It is important to remember that you do have other options. As you connect more with other people that you can trust (an AA sponsor might be one example), and with nondestructive things that comfort you, your need for self-destructive or self-harming activities will slowly diminish until one day it disappears.

Once you learn to establish safety and self-care in your present life, the work of understanding the past can begin.

Safety and Self-Care Diary

Please fill this out at home and take it to your individual therapy session if it would be helpful.

I do not take care of myself when . . .	Ways in which I do not take care of myself	I take good care of myself when . . .	Ways in which I take good care of myself	Supports in my life	New ways I can take care of myself
[example] I visit my family	Isolating	I talk to my friends	Exercising	My best friend	Join a therapy group

(continued)

The following questions and statements may help you think of ways to foster safety in your life and to care for yourself.

1. Have you ever felt safe? When?

_____

_____

_____

_____

_____

2. If I imagined feeling safe, I would imagine . . .

_____

_____

_____

_____

_____

3. The ways I take care of myself now include . . .

_____

_____

_____

_____

_____

4. The ways I don't take good enough care of myself include . . .

_____

_____

_____

_____

_____

(continued)

5. I take better care of myself when I am feeling . . .

_____

_____

_____

_____

_____

6. I fail to take care of myself when I am feeling . . .

_____

_____

_____

_____

7. People I do feel secure with and whom I consider using as supports are . . .

_____

_____

_____

_____

8. How would I ask one of those people if he or she could be there for me?

_____

_____

_____

_____

Session 3. Trust

In this worksheet, we are going to talk about how traumatic experiences affect the survivor's ability to trust herself, others, and the world around her. We also discuss the relationship between trust and self-blame and about the role that trust plays in recovery.

Trust is a basic human emotion. We grow up having to depend on and trust others from the day we are born. As infants, we are totally dependent on others to fulfill all of our basic needs. Being regularly and consistently attended to as infants and children instills a sense of trust in ourselves and our world. It allows us to feel that there is predictability and safety. When caregivers are able to provide this feeling *enough of the time,* the foundation is laid for a secure self and worldview. As we get older and become more competent, we can begin to do things for ourselves. The consistency and safety that we have already experienced in the world around us provide the basis for a growing sense of trust in ourselves and in other people.

When we encounter violence and cruelty, that sense of trust is betrayed. This is especially true if the people who hurt us are people whom we depended on for care and protection. If abuse began very early in your life, problems with trust may be very deeply felt. You may have learned that you could not trust the important people in your life to have your own best interests at heart. You may also have been told things like: "You don't deserve to be treated any better than this"; "This is the way to show love"; or "It is your fault that this is happening." Messages like these erode your ability to trust others and yourself.

If you were an adult when the violence occurred, your sense of security and trust in the world and your core beliefs that other people are safe can be shattered. You may no longer feel that it is safe to meet new people or to go out with friends. Alternatively, you may trust others too quickly and rush into relationships because being alone feels too overwhelming and frightening. Being too trusting can increase your risk of being hurt again.

Judgment and self-blame serve a purpose for many survivors. If you are an adult woman who was raped, self-blame may in some way help you feel more in control and give you the illusion of being able to prevent being raped in the future. If you were a child when you were abused, blaming yourself may have allowed you to stay connected to people you depended on or to feel that you could stop the abuse by behaving differently. Blaming yourself, therefore, can feel temporarily helpful. Over time, however, self-blame can make you feel like a bad person and erode your ability to trust yourself.

A major task of healing is learning how to judge situations and how to trust yourself and others in appropriate ways. This is not an easy thing to do. Often, survivors say that there is a part of them that wants to trust people, but that there is also a part of them that is terrified of trusting others. Beginning to trust others means opening yourself up to being disappointed or hurt. Letting others in may be a reminder that you didn't have the trusting relationships you deserved earlier in your life. You may never have admitted this to yourself before. It is a sad reality and very hard to accept. If you have been repeatedly betrayed by others, how can you risk trusting again? How can you tell if you can trust someone?

In order to build trust with others, it is important to take your time developing relationships and to take care of yourself in the process. For example, if you want to share something about yourself with a new friend, you could try saying, "I had a difficult childhood, and this sometimes affects how I feel today," without going into the details of your experience. You can then see how your friend reacts. Do

(continued)

you feel supported? Ignored? Understood? Dismissed? Did her reaction make you feel safer or more vulnerable? By taking your time and thinking about how the other person responds to you, you can get an idea of how much you can really trust this person. You can then decide how much you want to trust her in the future.

For many survivors, therapy provides a safe place where they can learn how to trust another person. Groups can be particularly helpful in developing trust, and perhaps that is partly why you are all here today. Slowly, you may find yourself trusting your therapist with more of the details and complexities of your life. You may develop a deeper and more compassionate understanding about why you don't always trust yourself. You can work with your therapist on rebuilding connections, gradually developing greater trust in others and in yourself. The following are statements that you can work on at home or bring to your therapist, as you continue to think about the issue of trust.

1. I think I can trust my ability to make good decisions when I (listen to my own needs, think through my decisions, etc.) . . .

_____

_____

_____

_____

_____

_____

2. I can trust myself at these times because I feel . . .

_____

_____

_____

_____

_____

3. I think I make bad decisions when I . . .

_____

_____

_____

_____

_____

_____

(continued)

4. I might be able to trust myself more if I asked myself (to slow down, do a "reality check," etc.) . . .

_____

_____

_____

_____

_____

5. I might be able to trust others more if I . . .

_____

_____

_____

_____

_____

_____

6. This week I will try to take better care of myself by . . .

_____

_____

_____

_____

_____

_____

Session 4. Remembering

In this worksheet, we are going to talk about the way in which traumatic experiences are stored in memory and the role of memory in the recovery process. Depending on your experience with remembering the traumatic events in your life, this worksheet may stir up some anxiety for you. We have found that remembering traumatic experiences is a difficult topic because it is often associated with an increase in posttraumatic stress symptoms. We want to reassure you that if these symptoms are triggered, it doesn't mean that you are "going crazy." Part of the purpose of today's worksheet is to explain why remembering is often associated with increased symptoms.

Memory is stored in many different ways. A young child who does not yet have the use of language stores memory through the senses of smell, touch, sight, and sound. Therefore, as adults, we may have no specific words for an early childhood memory, only a physical sensation that is vaguely associated with the past. As a child develops language, sensory memories become embedded in language and come to be stored and expressed in words. As adults, we retrieve and retell our memories as stories. A normal memory brings together the facts of the event, the emotions connected with the event, and the ways in which the event is part of one's larger life narrative. Ordinary memories evolve with time. As our sense of who we are in the world grows and changes, we may remember different aspects of the past, and the way we make sense of our experiences may grow and change as well.

Traumatic events disrupt normal memory. In moments of terror, people go into different states of consciousness that affect how the events are perceived and how they are stored in memory. There are two psychological concepts that are important to the understanding of traumatic memory and the impact of these memories on survivors: *flashbacks* and *dissociation*. Some people spontaneously go into a state of "fight or flight," while others enter a numbed state we call "dissociation." If during the trauma you felt your heart racing and your muscles tense, ready for "fight or flight," when you remember the event it may feel as though it is happening all over again. You may recall the sounds, the smells, or the imagery with an intensity that is similar to how you felt during the original trauma. This type of remembering is called a *flashback*. It can sometimes feel like a video or tape you can't shut off.

If, on the other hand, you reacted to the trauma by spontaneously going numb, or "spacing out," sometimes later on you may recall the facts without any emotion, as though they didn't really happen to you. Or you may be unable to remember part or all of the event in what is called *dissociative amnesia*. Some people experience this more than others.

At a later time, dissociated memories may be recalled in a splintered fashion. Memories of a traumatic experience may suddenly be "triggered" by a reminder of the original event. Sometimes we can tell why a memory is returning. You may be exposed to something that is obviously related to the traumatic experience: a smell, a place, or a person. At other times, the trigger is much less clear, everything in your life may seem to be going well—and, "out of nowhere," memories return. In fact, "things going well," including new relationships or new jobs, can be risky times for trauma survivors, who may unconsciously expect that they will get hurt again.

(continued)

The process of remembering traumatic experiences is often described as "confusing" or "crazy making." Survivors have said that remembering the past is like putting together a jigsaw puzzle: individual pieces don't mean much, but as they are slowly pieced together the picture begins to make sense. The feelings involved in remembering can be equally distressing. You may have the same feelings you had at the time of the experience, with an intensity that seems overwhelming. Similarly, many different feelings that were present at the time of the event can be reexperienced. These may include helplessness, powerlessness, rage, sadness, shame, and grief, to name a few. On the other hand, it may be very upsetting to some survivors to remember a traumatic experience in detail without any feeling whatsoever, and it may be frightening to be unable to remember part or all of the traumatic experience.

For some of you, remembering may have caused chaos in your life. Memories of traumatic events may intrude upon you at times when you least expect them and can make it hard to feel in control of your current responsibilities, such as work, parenting, and relationships. Emotions may be all out of proportion to what is going on in your present life. It is important to remind yourself when you are in the middle of the remembering process that it will pass. Eventually, the process can even be a valuable way for you to make new meaning out of your present-day life—which is, after all, why you are here in this group in the first place.

It is important to learn new ways to help yourself be more in control of the remembering process. Take flashbacks, for example. It may be helpful to remind yourself that a flashback is a piece of your history that is intruding from the past to the present. During a flashback, you may find it helpful to do things that make you feel less helpless. Remind yourself that you are not alone now and reach out to someone whom you can talk with, or just be with. Remind yourself that you are safe now; you are in the present and not in the past. Describe your present surroundings to yourself out loud. Press your feet against the floor or hold on to something that is comforting to you. Tighten and relax your fists or other muscles and focus on your breathing. Take three deep breaths. You have control over your body and can change the way it feels. Stand up. Turn on the light. Go for a walk. Get a hot cup of tea. Allow yourself to leave the memory alone until you are with someone with whom you can share your story. That person could be a close friend, an intimate partner, or possibly a therapist. When you can share your memories, you will feel less alone with them and can begin to work on making more sense of them.

Remembering is an ongoing process. It involves looking back and putting the pieces of one's life together, looking at what you already know in a different way, and starting to connect old feelings and images with words of your own. The healing process does not require remembering everything. What is most important is to understand the nature and impact of the trauma, in general, as well as the individual ways in which you learned to cope. You need a secure environment and new coping skills to start to recall things, both good and bad, that may have been forgotten for survival's sake. By working through the remembering process, you will come to develop a narrative for your life that feels cohesive and is meaningful to you. The following are questions and statements you can try to answer at home and bring to your individual therapist, if you wish.

(continued)

1. When I am under stress or feel overwhelmed I tend to (become confused, feel numb, get angry, etc.) . . .

_____

_____

_____

_____

_____

_____

_____

_____

2. When people ask me to talk about myself and my past, I realize that my memory starts at age _____. Other time spans that are sketchy include . . .

_____

_____

_____

_____

_____

_____

_____

3. I am aware that certain situations or interactions make me uncomfortable, such as . . .

_____

_____

_____

_____

_____

_____

_____

Until I understand the nature of this discomfort, I will minimize my involvement in these situations or seek support from others.

(continued)

4. I feel most comfortable when I am . . .

_____

_____

_____

_____

_____

_____

5. If I begin to have a flashback, I can help myself through it by (reminding myself that it is a memory, locating myself in my present immediate surroundings, exercising control over my body by tightening and relaxing muscles, etc.) . . .

_____

_____

_____

_____

_____

_____

_____

6. If I have a new memory and there is no one to share it with immediately, I can . . .

_____

_____

_____

_____

_____

_____

_____

Session 5. Shame and Self-Blame

Shame is a normal human feeling. We all feel ashamed at some time or other. We have all had moments of acute embarrassment when we feel foolish or self-conscious. Ordinary shame is a normal part of life. Though we've all felt acute shame at times, we learn that we can get over it because we know that there are other people who care for us and respect us. When we feel normal shame, it is a temporary feeling and allows us to feel that we can still be a good person, despite feeling silly or exposed.

Shame is different from guilt. Guilt is related to an action: we feel guilty when we've done something wrong. The way to relieve guilt is to take corrective action: to apologize and to make amends. But shame is about *who we are*. It is a very physical feeling that our bodies and our entire being are just wrong. Shame is a signal that something is not right in a relationship. It happens when we feel exposed, ridiculed, disrespected, or excluded. It is an intense feeling that makes us want to hide, "sink through the floor," or "crawl in a hole and die." The best way to relieve shame is to resist the impulse to hide and instead to connect with people who care about us. Shared, spontaneous laughter is the best antidote to shame. It signals to us that we are accepted for *who we are,* that we belong.

How we grow up influences how we develop and manage feelings of shame. When adults correct the behavior of a child without blaming the child for who he or she is, the child can learn to behave differently without losing his or her sense of self. But if we have grown up without that secure feeling of being cared for and respected, we can develop destructive shame. When adults treat children abusively, children begin to identify with a feeling of inner "badness." Instead of experiencing transient feelings of self-consciousness or embarrassment, children develop chronic feelings of self-loathing. They come to feel dirty, humiliated, and defiled.

Self-blame also develops in situations in which abused or neglected children begin to feel responsible for the actions of others. An abused child will often say to him- or herself, "I am bad. That must be why my parents hurt me." There are a number of reasons why a child might develop this belief. Sometimes the parent actually blames the child directly, saying, "This is your fault." Sometimes blame may be implied in more subtle and nonverbal ways. Self-blame is also a way for the child to make sense out of something that is otherwise difficult, if not impossible, to understand. For example, it is easier to think "If I wasn't so terrible, my parents wouldn't get so angry and hurt me" than to wonder "What's wrong with my parents that they get so angry and lose control?"

Taking responsibility may also seem to give a sense of control, although that control is only an illusion. Blaming oneself for the inexcusable behavior of others deepens feelings of shame. These feelings often last long into adulthood.

Destructive shame may also develop when the child believes that he or she has encouraged or participated in hurtful behavior. Even though the child is being hurt or violated, he or she may feel a special connection to the abusive adult. An abusive encounter may have been the only time that child receives what seemed like positive attention, rather than being ignored or yelled at. Or perhaps the child's body physiologically responded to how he or she was being touched. Sometimes a child is violated repeatedly before he or she realizes that what is happening is wrong.

(continued)

Adult victims of sexual assault may also feel destructive shame and self-blame, especially when they are ostracized and shamed by the people who matter to them. They may be regarded as "sluts" because of what they wore when they were out in public or because they were drinking. Even survivors of rape in wartime may sometimes be shunned by their own communities, regarded as "dirty" or "damaged goods," and suspected of allowing what happened or not fighting hard enough. When this happens, it is all too easy for survivors themselves to feel "dirty."

Regardless of the circumstances, **it is never the victim's fault that she or he was hurt or violated.** Letting go of self-blame allows survivors to begin the grieving process that is so essential to the development of a healthy sense of self-respect. This grieving process allows survivors to feel the sadness of their lives without reliving it or denying it. By accepting the sadness and hurt as parts of their past, survivors no longer have the need to protect themselves from the crippling effects of self-blame.

You can let go of destructive shame. Recognize when you are feeling it, and learn how to protect yourself from it. Find someone trustworthy to talk to and get support. Your confidant could be a family member, friend, partner, or therapist. The important point is that you have come to trust that this is a person who cares for you and respects you. It always feels risky to talk about things you feel ashamed of. You may fear that your confidant will be disgusted by you, think less of you, or even abandon you. But as you share more and discover that this doesn't happen, you may be surprised at how much better you feel.

There are many benefits to talking about feelings of shame and self-blame. You may feel less separate from people, improve your relationships, and become more self-compassionate. Sometimes survivors feel that only the abuser knows her "inner badness," and talking about this may reduce your shameful "bond" with the person who abused you (Cloitre et al., 2006). You can find a trusted person who will accept you as you are, with all of your shameful secrets. This can begin with your individual therapist or with another person who has been consistently trustworthy and supportive. Remember to be compassionate to yourself and recognize your own courage as you begin throwing off the burden of shame.

Please fill out this worksheet at home and take it to your individual therapist if it would be helpful.

1. When thinking about shame you have experienced, which experiences have reflected ordinary shame (↑) and which have reflected destructive shame (↓)?

(continued)

2. Remember that when feeling destructive shame, people are often judging and blaming themselves for the actions of others who were more powerful. In the left column, think of words you have used in the past to judge and blame yourself. On the right, think of new ways to understand what happened to you in the past.

(continued)

3. The ways I try to protect myself from feelings of destructive shame include . . .

_____

_____

_____

_____

_____

_____

_____

_____

_____

4. Replacing negative judgments about oneself with kinder thoughts often helps. What are some positive words you could use to describe yourself?

_____

_____

_____

_____

_____

_____

_____

_____

_____

_____

Session 6. Compassion

Since you have joined this group, you have all focused on the complexity of your emotions and on the difficulty in understanding why certain feelings are evoked in particular situations. You have also focused on how similar many of your emotional experiences are, particularly in the areas of shame and self-blame. Throughout the course of the group you have expressed feelings of compassion toward other group members and offered them support and encouragement. Many of you have observed how hard it is to feel these same compassionate feelings about yourselves.

The word *compassion* comes from the Latin word for suffering. It means "deep awareness of the suffering of another or of oneself, along with a desire to alleviate it." When you feel compassion for another person, you experience caring and empathy for the other person's pain. Turning this compassionate lens toward yourself can feel like a real challenge. However, having compassion for yourself is not really all that different from having compassion for others. When one can be self-compassionate, feelings of shame are eased and they can slowly change into kindness toward the self. Self-compassion reminds us that we are all human and helps us be less judgmental about our perceived defects.

When someone is suffering, we do not, as a rule, tell them that they need to be perfect or make their suffering worse by criticizing them. Ask yourself why you believe that you do not deserve the same tolerance and understanding that you give to others. It is hard to have self-compassion if you believe that you should be perfect. For people who have grown up in abusive settings, it is not uncommon to feel defective, unlovable, and deserving of mistreatment. Sometimes we imagine that if we had only been better we might have been loved and cared for, and we blame ourselves harshly for failing to live up to impossible standards of perfection. We tell ourselves things like "I'm so stupid" or "I should have known better." One way to help improve self-esteem and increase compassion for ourselves is to notice this kind of negative self-talk and to try replacing it with a more balanced perspective. We can take pride in our strengths and forgive our weaknesses, accepting the fact that we are only human. In this way, we may begin to move away from impossible expectations of perfection and move toward accepting ourselves as we are.

Survivors may also cope with feeling helpless by wanting to "do something." Action can at times feel satisfying, whether that action is healthy or not. At times action can relieve pain in a productive way. For example, an action as simple as taking a walk can soothe anxiety and help reestablish a more grounded feeling. Other actions, however, although initially soothing, can be harmful later on. Substance abuse and other forms of self-destructive behavior are common examples. Many survivors also describe themselves as wanting to "do something" for others. They may characterize themselves as "people pleasers," wanting to make things better for others. Although compassion can involve action, it does not necessarily have to. Compassion often means simply being present: sitting, listening, and accepting the person in her pain without trying to fix it. As you offer compassion to others, you will learn that just being there can help. Self-compassion requires a similar acceptance of yourself and your pain. A harsh stance never helps anyone to grow and heal. Learning to have a compassionate perspective is an important part of healing and recovery.

During your time in the group you have come to know each other and feel respect and compassion for each other. Can you offer this compassion to yourself as well?

(continued)

Alternatively, you may wish to put together a list of Personal Rights, or things that you are entitled to do. These may include the right to:

1. Make mistakes.
2. Change your mind.
3. Express both negative and positive feelings.
4. Say "I don't understand" or "I don't know."
5. Spend time the way you choose.
6. Not have to explain yourself.
7. Be listened to.
8. Be your own judge.
9. Be your own champion.
10. Live in peace.

Compassion Homework Exercises

1. When I feel judgmental and critical toward myself, here are some of the things I say to myself:

_____

_____

_____

_____

_____

_____

_____

_____

_____

_____

2. When I am feeling compassionate toward others, here are some of the things I say to them:

_____

_____

_____

_____

_____

(continued)

_____

_____

_____

_____

_____

3. Do I deserve the same compassion and kindness as other people do? If not, why not? Where did these beliefs come from?

_____

_____

_____

_____

_____

_____

_____

_____

_____

_____

4. If I imagined feeling self-compassion, what are some of the things I could say to myself?

_____

_____

_____

_____

_____

_____

_____

_____

_____

Session 7. Anger

Anger is often thought of as a negative emotion. Women in particular are taught to shy away from anger and its expression. As women, we have been taught that anger is "unattractive" and "unladylike." There are some injustices, however, that make all of us angry, and it is important to redefine anger as a useful and at times a positive emotion.

Anger is a natural response to being victimized and abused. If you do not allow yourself to be aware of your anger, you may turn it inward or misdirect it against others. Anger turned inward can manifest in many unhealthy ways, including depression, substance abuse, self-injurious behaviors, self-hatred, or even physical illness. Anger turned outward can be expressed by intense or misdirected rage at people who are not the true source of your distress. Sometimes survivors describe with sadness that it is the safe and loving people in their lives who are the recipients of their anger. Other survivors describe not having an "intensity dial" as it relates to anger, but having only an on-and-off switch. They report that when they feel their anger, it is always with the same intensity, regardless of the situation.

Many trauma survivors are fearful about allowing themselves to recognize and explore their anger. It is not uncommon to hear survivors say that they are afraid that once they open that floodgate they will be unable to close it. Some fear that, if they become angry, they would be as bad as the people who abused them. Survivors may share that they have never seen a healthy expression of anger.

One way to make angry feelings less frightening is to remember that anger is just a feeling, and is not necessarily something that needs to be acted upon. The fantasy of how you would choose to express your anger can be just that—a fantasy, not an action plan. When you allow yourself to imagine taking revenge on the people who harmed you, killing them, hurting them, or exposing them, these are only thoughts, not rageful behaviors. Allowing these thoughts in can help you direct your anger away from yourself and toward the aggressor, where it belongs.

It is also important to recognize that there is a big difference between helpless rage and righteous indignation. Rage is what people feel when they are powerless to protect themselves against violence and domination. Righteous indignation can be a source of positive action to protect yourself and others. It can be a powerful antidote to the misery of helpless rage.

Allowing oneself to explore one's anger requires self-confidence. Being angry means recognizing that you are worth something and did not deserve the treatment that you received. It holds the abusive person responsible for his actions and frees you to live with less self-hatred and self-blame. Being angry can also motivate you to help others who are similarly hurt. When you join with others to resist and repair injustice, you become part of a group dedicated to making a better world. We call this a "survivor mission."

A concept related to anger is forgiveness. Oftentimes victims of injustice are told that they must "let go" of their anger so that they can forgive the perpetrator. However, there is no evidence that this is necessary for all survivors. Forgiving the people who harmed you is not a requirement of healing.

Forgiveness often occurs spontaneously when perpetrators acknowledge the harm they have done, express sincere remorse, and offer to try to make amends. It is a beautiful thing when this happens, but unfortunately it happens only rarely. In the absence of a sincere apology, it is difficult for survivors to transcend righteous anger.

(continued)

The only forgiveness necessary in the healing process is forgiveness for yourself, for all the ways that you may have mistakenly held yourself responsible for the abuse. Having compassion for ourselves can best occur when we can better identify and explore our anger.

Anger Homework Exercises

1. Things that make me angry include . . .

_____

_____

_____

_____

_____

2. When I feel angry, I . . .

_____

_____

_____

_____

_____

3. Unhealthy ways I express my anger include . . .

_____

_____

_____

_____

_____

4. New ways I can imagine expressing my anger include . . .

_____

_____

_____

_____

_____

Session 8. Self-Image/Body Image

Newborn infants are full of movement. Through bodily motion, infants explore their world and express their first emotions. Through physical contact with a soothing person, they learn to go from a state of excitement or fear to one of calm. As children grow, their relationship with their bodies develops according to their physical health and what they learn from their family and the wider society they live in.

In our society, a great deal of attention is paid to how we look. TV ads and magazines bombard women with images of perfect hair, flawless complexions, and slender, shapely figures dressed so as to appeal to men and to a certain ideal. Men are bombarded with ads defining product-driven sex appeal with images of rippling muscles and implied strength. When self-esteem begins to be based on having or getting these supposedly ideal physical attributes, it is difficult not to feel inadequate, self-conscious, or unsure of oneself. An antidote to this constant cultural messaging is for children, early in their lives, to experience steady affection and appreciation for who they are. Later in life, such nurturing will help these children be less vulnerable to basing self-esteem on physical appearance.

However, when children's bodies have been violated, exposed to the threat of harm, or exploited sexually, the physical self often becomes an object of fear or disgust. Survivors may feel that their bodies are bad or unclean. They may either try to ignore their bodies, at one extreme, or become preoccupied with their internal bodily sensations at the other. Some survivors avoid getting needed dental or medical care; others may seek medical attention repeatedly for symptoms that don't seem to have a medical explanation. Survivors may feel asexual and try to minimize their sexual identity by dressing in clothing that hides their shape. They might withdraw from interpersonal relationships that involve physical intimacy. Other reactions can be quite the opposite. Some survivors may become flirtatious, provocative, or even sexually promiscuous as a way of feeling powerful. Others may use their sexuality to obtain a brief respite from feeling alone and unloved.

If survivors have felt that their bodies have betrayed them, they may also exert great efforts to control them. They might groom themselves obsessively. They may feel safe only when feeling in complete control of what goes in and out of their bodies through restrictive dieting or bingeing and purging of food. They may also feel that through self-induced physical pain, such as cutting, they might have increased control over their feelings and emotions.

A fear of being in one's body affects health care, relatedness to others, self-esteem, and self-confidence. Many assault survivors have reported struggles with disordered eating and a dislike or hatred for their bodies. These issues create symptoms often needing medical care, but leave the survivor hesitant to seek it out. Some survivors have shared that they have found it helpful to let medical providers know how difficult it can feel to allow another person to touch them or to see them undressed.

Fear of being in the body can also extend to feelings about pregnancy, childbirth, and child care. Body changes in pregnancy can evoke strong fears of one's body being out of control. Caring for children can evoke intensely emotional and physical memories of one's own childhood. It is important to have safe places to talk about the impacts of trauma on all aspects of self-image and body image.

An important task in the healing process is the establishment of a positive regard for one's physical self. The following are statements and questions to consider in order to become more familiar

(continued)

with messages you received about your body as a child and the ways in which you can begin to establish a healing relationship with your body as an adult.

1. When I was a child, I enjoyed the following physical activities:

   _____

   _____

   _____

   _____

2. As a child, the messages I learned about my body were:

   _____

   _____

   _____

   _____

3. I take care of my physical self in these ways:

   _____

   _____

   _____

   _____

4. I could take better care of myself if I . . .

   _____

   _____

   _____

   _____

5. A list of questions I would like to ask my doctor includes:

   _____

   _____

   _____

   _____

Session 9. Relationships with and Connections to Others

As much as we might like to think of ourselves as self-sufficient, we depend on others in every aspect of our lives. We are social beings from birth. As infants and young children, we are totally dependent on our caregivers. If those caregivers were predictable and trustworthy and treated us with loving care, we develop what psychologists call *secure attachment*. Our caregivers provide us with a "safe base" from which we can gradually learn to explore the larger world. Secure attachment in early life becomes the foundation for mutually trustworthy and satisfying relationships in adult life.

However, for people whose trust has been repeatedly betrayed, relationships with others can be quite difficult and complicated. Abuse survivors, as adults, are likely to bring expectations from what they learned in their earliest relationships to their current relationships, even in everyday social interactions. Survivors may expect to be mistreated and may react as if the very same things that happened in the past were happening in the present. Sometimes just a slight similarity to someone from the past—a tone of voice, a scent, a habit of some sort—can cause a survivor to have such a reaction.

We all need people in our lives, for validation, support, and companionship. Risking connection is complicated and leaves open the possibility of disappointment and heartache, but the other option, to stay in total disconnect, is painful as well. If children have grown up with terrible secrets, they may fear letting anyone get to know them very well, and so may continue leading a very constricted personal life into adulthood. Many survivors, who have participated in past groups, have cited loneliness as one of the most painful effects of their trauma histories. They have expressed a great fear of letting others get to know them well. If they have taken risks and been disappointed, these survivors often blamed themselves.

If personal boundaries were poorly defined or frequently violated in childhood, adult survivors may find it hard to separate their own feelings from those of others. For example, one parent might have inappropriately confided in the child about problems with the other parent, such as emotional difficulties or financial troubles. Such neediness in caregivers can overwhelm and confuse a child or make the child feel that the only way to *get* any care is to try and *give* care to the adult. Such "care" given by a child might have included participating in sexual intimacy. In adulthood, the pattern of exchanging emotional support and/or sex for some sense of protection or security may persist, even if the survivor does not really want to be with a partner or is being mistreated by that partner.

When abuse goes unrecognized by others, children can learn to minimize, deny, or confuse their experience. They might learn to do this so completely that in later relationships, even in ones that really are safe, they experience their own true emotions as threatening.

Many adult survivors of childhood abuse find themselves repeatedly entering into relationships with abusive partners for many reasons. One is that survivors have not learned the skills they need in order to tell whether a potential partner is safe. Some survivors wonder whether their vulnerability can somehow be sensed by others. Others wonder whether a relationship in which they are controlled or victimized is somehow the only kind of relationship they know how to have or feel that they deserve.

When you have been traumatized, it is important to learn to identify what is safe and worthy of your time and attention. In relationships this can be done by **asking questions and clarifying intent**—finding out, for example, what another person means by a facial expression, a gesture, or a

(continued)

statement that seems unclear. Doing so can feel awkward or scary at first, particularly because the whole idea of being allowed to ask questions is often unfamiliar to survivors. But it is upon these direct communications that solid relationships can be built and unhealthy relationships can sometimes be avoided. One gradually "tests the waters," trying to keep in mind that each situation is truly new and one is not doomed to repeat the past.

The following questions are designed to help you think about your connections to others and the ways in which you can help yourself feel increasingly safe and secure in those connections.

1. Who are the people in my life with whom I feel most connected?

_____

_____

_____

_____

_____

_____

_____

_____

_____

_____

2. How am I most comfortable socially (one on one, in groups, in AA, etc.)?

_____

_____

_____

_____

_____

_____

_____

_____

_____

(continued)

3. Are there repeating patterns in relationships that cause me discomfort? Can I trace any of these patterns to expectations I bring from my past?

_____

_____

_____

_____

_____

_____

_____

_____

_____

_____

_____

4. What can I do when someone does not respect my boundaries or my feelings?

_____

_____

_____

_____

_____

_____

_____

_____

_____

_____

_____

Session 10. Making Meaning of the Past and the Process of Recovery

Traumatized people are likely to feel unsafe in their day-to-day lives as a result of what they have experienced in their past. As we have seen throughout these sessions, some of the behaviors survivors use to cope (avoidance, clinging to others, risk taking of various kinds, self-harm, alcohol or drug use, eating disorders) can develop into sources of embarrassment, as can emotional reactions such as fearfulness, numbness, dissociation, and explosive anger. These aftereffects can contribute to feeling abnormal or out of control.

As we have discussed, the first priority in any recovery process is to restore a sense of safety and control. Take a close look at your everyday life and pay attention to any of the ways that your personal and emotional safety is at risk. Present-day safety must be established before trying to think too deeply about the traumas of the past. If one is using drugs or alcohol to control feelings, it is important to get clean and sober and to learn to cope in ways that are not self-destructive. The same is true for self-harming (e.g., cutting or burning), reckless driving, eating poorly, binge eating and/or purging, or being in relationships that place one in physical or emotional danger. Healthy regulation of bodily functions, such as sleep and exercise, are essential as well. Not to be overlooked are financial and housing security. Many survivors say that they get useful help from support groups, 12-step programs, and group and individual psychotherapies.

Finding healthy coping strategies that help you relax and clear your mind is an important part of recovery. Such strategies often include focusing attention on one or more of the senses in the present moment and might include deep breathing exercises, visualization, or other forms of meditation. Sometimes psychiatric medications, appropriately prescribed, can also be a great help in restoring an inner sense of control over symptoms.

The focus on establishing safety allows time for trust to build within therapy relationships, as well as within outside relationships. This is a time when one can be developing a new or renewed sense of competency, mastery, and increased self-esteem. One can work on becoming more practiced in talking about oneself, learning to control one's feelings, and experiencing them in the middle ranges rather than in the "all-or-nothing" extremes.

As healthy strategies for coping and problem solving in the present become more reliably established, talking about past traumatic experiences can begin at a pace that is safe—and not retraumatizing—for each individual person. In this way, survivors can begin to reconnect feelings to events, place them in context, and give them meaning.

Within a trusting relationship, survivors can break their silence and share their secrets. For many, this may be the first time they are able to share parts of their history without feeling either numb and emotionally constricted or overwhelmed. Sharing one's history allows for a more complete understanding of the past. This understanding can bring with it deep sadness, as you begin to appreciate all that you have been through. Growth occurs as you realize that while you can never change the past, you do have the ability to change the present and to take more control of your life. As you do this, the effects of the past will lessen. Over time, the current impact of the trauma diminishes, so that it no longer feels like the center of your life.

With this understanding comes the capacity to think about the future, to make plans, and to realize ambitions. This is often a time to reconnect with others, as you realize that you have something

(continued)

to offer them. Many survivors choose to be sponsors in 12-step programs, to become politically active, or to volunteer services to those less fortunate. Others contribute in less visible, but equally important, ways. Although we have talked in these sessions about all the ways in which survivors may *not* see the world clearly, there are other ways in which it is very hard to fool them. This may be a unique strength belonging to the survivors of all injustices.

Making Meaning of the Past

Making meaning of a traumatic experience is a very complicated challenge and something that takes time. We give meaning to events to make them comprehensible, and the way we do this is often based on how we view ourselves and the world. Is this a world in which bad things happen to good people? Or do we believe bad things happen because we deserve them? Do you believe in God or have a spiritual faith? Is there some greater connection between events, or is each event separate and only related to other events by coincidence? Whatever your belief system is, it provides a context with which to understand your life.

Our belief systems, and how we answer such questions, usually have a lot to do with the belief system we grew up with. As we have seen, we take what we have learned in the past into the rest of our lives, often unconsciously expecting the same kinds of events and relationships even in very new and potentially different circumstances. Sometimes these expectations have a way of making the familiar patterns repeat themselves.

Recovery and meaning making evolve over time. Making meaning of the past involves understanding the world of the child from a new perspective—your perspective as an adult standing outside the abusive situation. It often involves grieving for the past that actually happened, but also for the loss of the past that one wishes one had. Through development of compassion for one's past and present self, growth occurs. For every member of this group, we hope that this experience will help you with this process and with letting yourself have a more gentle and self-caring appreciation of yourself and the ways you have coped. Completing this group is an achievement and a further step in your recovery. Allow yourself to appreciate what you have accomplished, and know that you have the strength and resilience to continue this important and affirming work.

1. Some of the ways I have tried to protect myself from being hurt include . . .

_____

_____

_____

_____

_____

_____

_____

_____

(continued)

2. Some of the ways of self-protection that are actually harmful or place me at further risk include . . .

_____

_____

_____

_____

_____

_____

_____

3. Ways I can begin to express a fuller range of feelings include . . .

_____

_____

_____

_____

_____

_____

_____

4. Ways I can take action to change things for the better include . . .

_____

_____

_____

_____

_____

_____

References

Aldrich, H., & Kallivayalil, D. (2013). The impact of homicide on survivors and clinicians. *Journal of Loss and Trauma, 18*(4), 362–377.

Armeni, D. T. (2014, May 11). A soldier fights off the cold. *New York Times*, p. SR11.

Bateman, A. W., & Fonagy, P. (2004). Mentalization-based treatment of BPD. *Journal of Personality Disorders, 18*(1), 36–51.

Bernard, H. S., & Mackenzie, K. R. (Eds.). (1994). *Basics of group psychotherapy.* New York: Guilford Press.

Bradley, R. G., & Follingstad, D. R. (2003). Group therapy for incarcerated women who experienced interpersonal violence: A pilot study. *Journal of Traumatic Stress, 16*, 337–340.

Briere, J., & Jordan, C. E. (2009). Childhood maltreatment, intervening variables, and adult psychological difficulties in women: An overview. *Trauma, Violence, and Abuse, 10*(4), 375–388.

Briere, J., & Rickards, S. (2007). Self-awareness, affect regulation, and relatedness: Differential sequels of childhood versus adult victimization experiences. *Journal of Nervous and Mental Disease, 195*(6), 497–503.

Brown, D. (2009). Assessment of attachment and abuse history and adult attachment style. In C. A. Courtois & J. D. Ford (Eds.), *Treating complex traumatic stress disorders: An evidence-based guide* (pp. 124–144). New York: Guilford Press.

Brown, N., Kallivayalil, D., & Harvey, M. (2012). Braiding of resilience and psychopathology in the narratives of trauma survivors in early recovery. *Psychological Trauma: Theory, Research, Practice, and Policy, 4*(1), 102–111.

Carroll, L. (2011). *Alice's adventures in wonderland.* Peterborough, Canada: Broadview Press.

Chard, K. (2005). An evaluation of cognitive processing therapy for the treatment of posttraumatic stress disorder related to childhood sexual abuse. *Journal of Clinical and Consulting Psychology, 73*, 965–971.

Charuvastra, A., & Cloitre, M. (2008). Social bonds and posttraumatic stress disorder. *Annual Review of Psychology, 59*, 301–328.

Classen, C., Koopman, C., Nevill-Manning, K., & Spiegel, D. (2001). A preliminary report comparing trauma-focused and present-focused group therapy against waitlisted condition among childhood sexual abuse survivors with PTSD. *Journal of Aggression, Maltreatment, and Trauma, 4*, 265–288.

Classen, C., Palesh, O., & Aggarwal, R. (2005). Sexual revictimization: A review of the empirical literature. *Trauma, Violence and Abuse, 6*, 103–129.

Cloitre, M., Courtois, C. A., Ford, J. D., Green, B. L., Alexander, P., Briere, J., et al. (2012). The ISTSS expert consensus treatment guidelines for complex PTSD in adults. Retrieved from *www.istss.org*.

Cloitre, M., Cohen, L. R., & Koenen, K. C. (2006). *Treating survivors of childhood abuse: Psychotherapy for the interrupted life.* New York: Guilford Press.

Cloitre, M., & Koenen, K. C. (2001). The impact of borderline personality disorder on process group outcome among women with posttraumatic stress disorder related to childhood abuse. *International Journal of Group Psychotherapy, 51,* 379–398.

Cloitre, M., Miranda, R., Stovall-McClough, K. C., & Han, H. (2005). Beyond PTSD: Emotion regulation and interpersonal problems as predictors of functional impairment in survivors of childhood abuse. *Behavior Therapy, 36*(2), 119–124.

Courtois, C. A., & Ford, J. D. (Eds.). (2009). *Treating complex traumatic stress disorders: An evidence-based guide.* New York: Guilford Press.

Courtois, C. A., Ford, J. D., & Cloitre, M. (2009). Best practices in psychotherapy for adults. In C. A. Courtois & J. D. Ford (Eds.), *Treating complex traumatic stress disorders: An evidence-based guide* (pp. 82–103). New York: Guilford Press.

DeLucia-Waack, J. L., & Fauth, J. (2004). Effective supervision of group leaders. In J. L. DeLucia-Waack, D. A. Gerrity, C. R. Kalodner, & M. T. Riva (Eds.), *Handbook of group counseling and psychotherapy* (pp. 136–150). Thousand Oaks, CA: Sage.

Desai, R. A., Harpaz-Rotem, I., Najavits, L. M., & Rosenheck, R. A. (2008). Impact of the Seeking Safety program on clinical outcomes among homeless female veterans with psychiatric disorders. *Psychiatric Services, 59*(9), 996–1003.

Dunn, N. J., Rehm, L. P., Schillaci, J., Souchek, J., Mehta, P., Ashton, C. M., et al. (2007). A randomized trial of self-management and psychoeducational group therapies for comorbid chronic posttraumatic stress disorder and depressive disorder. *Journal of Traumatic Stress, 20*(3), 221–237.

Fallot, R. D., & Harris, M. (2002). The Trauma Recovery and Empowerment Model (TREM): Conceptual and practical issues in a group intervention for women. *Community Mental Health Journal, 38*(6), 475–485.

Fallot, R. D., McHugo, G. J., Harris, M., & Xie, H. (2011). The trauma recovery and empowerment model: A quasi-experimental effectiveness study. *Journal of Dual Diagnosis, 7*(1–2), 74–89.

Felitti, V. J., Anda, R. F., Nordenberg, D., Williamson, D. F., Spitz, A. M., Edwards, V., et al. (1998). Relationship of childhood abuse and household dysfunction to many of the leading causes of death in adults: The Adverse Childhood Experiences (ACE) Study. *American Journal of Preventive Medicine, 14*(4), 245–258.

Foa, E. B., Keane, T. M., Friedman, M. J., & Cohen, J. A. (Eds.). (2009). *Effective treatments for PTSD: Practice guidelines from the International Society for Traumatic Stress Studies* (2nd ed.). New York: Guilford Press.

Fonagy, P., & Target, M. (2002). Early intervention and the development of self-regulation. *Psychoanalytic Inquiry, 22*(3), 307–335.

Fonagy, P., Target, M., Gergely, G., Allen, J. G., & Bateman, A. W. (2003). The developmental roots of borderline personality disorder in early attachment relationships: A theory and some evidence. *Psychoanalytic Inquiry, 23*(3), 412–459.

Ford, J. D., & Russo, E. (2006). Trauma-focused, present-centered, emotional self-regulation approach to integrated treatment for posttraumatic stress and addiction: Trauma adaptive recovery group education and therapy (TARGET). *American Journal of Psychotherapy, 60*(4), 335–355.

Ford, J. D., Steinberg, K. L., & Zhang, W. (2011). A randomized clinical trial comparing affect regulation and social problem-solving psychotherapies for mothers with victimization-related PTSD. *Behavior Therapy, 42*(4), 560–578.

Foy, D., Glynn, S., Schnurr, P., Jankowski, M., Wattenberg, M., Weiss, D., et al. (2000). Group therapy. In E. B. Foa, T. M. Keane, & M. J. Friedman (Eds.), *Effective treatments for PTSD: Practice guidelines from the International Society for Traumatic Stress Studies* (pp. 155–175). New York: Guilford Press.

Frisman, L., Ford, J., Lin, H. J., Mallon, S., & Chang, R. (2008). Outcomes of trauma treatment using the TARGET model. *Journal of Groups in Addiction and Recovery, 3*(3–4), 285–303.

Fritch, A. M., & Lynch, S. M. (2008). Group treatment for adult survivors of interpersonal trauma. *Journal of Psychological Trauma, 7*(3), 145–169.

Harned, M. S., & Linehan, M. M. (2008). Integrating dialectical behavior therapy and prolonged exposure to treat co-occurring borderline personality disorder and PTSD: Two case studies. *Cognitive and Behavioral Practice, 15*(3), 263–276.

Harney, P. A., & Harvey, M. R. (1999). Group psychotherapy: An overview. In B. Young & D. Blake (Eds.), *Group treatments for post traumatic stress disorder* (pp. 1–13). New York: Brunner/Mazel.

Harris, M. (1998). *T.R.E.M. Trauma Recovery and Empowerment: A clinician's guide to working with women in groups.* New York: Free Press.

Harvey, M. R. (1996). An ecological view of psychological trauma and trauma recovery. *Journal of Traumatic Stress, 9*(1), 3–23.

Harvey, M. R., & Tummala-Narra, P. (Eds.). (2007). *Sources and expressions of resiliency in trauma survivors: Ecological theory, multicultural practice.* Binghamton, NY: Haworth Maltreatment & Trauma Press.

Hazzard, A., Rogers, J. H., & Angert, L. (1993). Factors affecting group therapy outcome for adult sexual abuse survivors. *International Journal of Group Psychotherapy, 434*, 453–468.

Herman, J. L. (1992). Complex PTSD: A syndrome in survivors of prolonged and repeated trauma. *Journal of Traumatic Stress, 5*, 377–391.

Herman, J. L. (2015). *Trauma and recovery.* New York: Basic Books. (Original work published 1992)

Herman, J. L., Perry, J. C., & van der Kolk, B. A. (1989). Childhood trauma in borderline personality disorder. *American Journal of Psychiatry, 146*, 490–495.

Hien, D. A., Cohen, L. R., Miele, G. M., Litt, L. C., & Capstick, C. (2004). Promising treatments for women with comorbid PTSD and substance use disorders. *American Journal of Psychiatry, 161*(8), 1426–1432.

Klein, R. H., & Schermer, V. L. (Eds.). (2000). *Group psychotherapy for psychological trauma.* New York: Guilford Press.

Liotti, G. (2004). Trauma, dissociation, and disorganized attachment: Three strands of a single braid. *Psychotherapy: Theory, Research, Practice, Training, 41*, 472–486.

Lubin, H., & Johnson, D. (2008). *Trauma-centered group psychotherapy for women: A clinician's manual.* Philadelphia: Haworth Press.

Lubin, J., Loris, M., Burt, J., & Johnson, D. R. (1998). Efficacy of psychoeducational group therapy in reducing symptoms of posttraumatic stress disorder among multiply traumatized women. *American Journal of Psychiatry, 155*, 1172–1177.

Lynch, T. R., Trost, W. T., Salsman, N., & Linehan, M. M. (2007). Dialectical behavior therapy for borderline personality disorder. *Annual Review of Clinical Psychology, 3*, 181–205.

Mendelsohn, M., Herman, J. L., Schatzow, E., Levitan, J., Kallivayalil, D., & Coco, M. (2011). *The Trauma Recovery Group: A guide for practitioners.* New York: Guilford Press.

Najavits, L. M. (2002). *Seeking Safety: A treatment manual for PTSD and substance abuse.* New York: Guilford Press.

Najavits, L. M., Weiss, R. D., Shaw, S. R., & Muenz, L. R. (1998). "Seeking Safety": Outcome of a new cognitive-behavioral psychotherapy for women with posttraumatic stress disorder and substance dependence. *Journal of Traumatic Stress, 11*(3), 437–456.

Parten, M., & Newhall, S. (1943). Social behavior of preschool children. In R. Barker, J. Kounin, & H. Wright (Eds.), *Child behavior and development: A course of representative studies* (pp. 509–525). New York: McGraw-Hill.

Pearlman, L. A., & Courtois, C. A. (2005). Clinical applications of the attachment framework: Relational treatment of complex trauma. *Journal of Traumatic Stress, 18*(5), 449–459.

Ray, R. D., & Webster, R. (2010). Group interpersonal psychotherapy for veterans with posttraumatic stress disorder: A pilot study. *International Journal of Group Psychotherapy, 60*(1), 131–140.

Rutan, J. S., Stone, W. N., & Shay, J. J. (2007). *Psychodynamic group psychotherapy* (4th ed.). New York: Guilford Press.

Saakvitne, K. W., Gamble, S., Pearlman, L. A., & Lev, B. T. (2000). *Risking connection: A training curriculum for working with survivors of childhood abuse.* Baltimore: Sidran Press.

Salsman, N., & Linehan, M. M. (2006). Dialectical-behavioral therapy for borderline personality disorder. *Primary Psychiatry, 13*(5), 51–58.

Salston, M., & Figley, C. R. (2003). Secondary traumatic stress effects of working with survivors of criminal victimization. *Journal of Traumatic Stress, 16*(2), 167–174.

Schnurr, P., Friedman, M., Foy, D., Shea, M., Hsieh, F. Lavori, P., et al. (2003). Randomized trial of trauma-focused group therapy for posttraumatic stress disorder: Results from a Department of Veterans Affairs Cooperative Study. *Archives of General Psychiatry, 60,* 481–489.

Sewell, K. W., & Williams, A. M. (2001). Construing stress: A constructivist therapeutic approach to post-traumatic stress reactions. In R. A. Niemeyer (Ed.), *Meaning reconstruction and the experience of loss* (pp. 293–310). Washington, DC: American Psychological Association.

Shea, M. T., McDevitt-Murphy, M., Ready, D. J., & Schnurr, P. P. (2009). Group therapy. In E. B. Foa, T. M. Keane, M. J. Friedman, & J. A. Cohen (Eds.), *Effective treatments for PTSD: Practice guidelines from the International Society for Traumatic Stress Studies* (2nd ed., pp. 306–326). New York: Guilford Press.

Sinozich, S., & Langton, L. (2014). *Rape and sexual assault victimization among college-age females, 1995–2013.* Washington, DC: U.S. Department of Justice, Office of Justice Programs, Bureau of Justice Statistics.

Sloan, D., & Beck, G. (2016). Group treatment for PTSD. *PTSD Research Quarterly, 27*(2), 1–9.

Sloan, D. M., Feinstein, B. A., Gallagher, M. W., Beck, J. G., & Keane, T. M. (2013). Efficacy of group treatment for posttraumatic stress disorder symptoms: A meta-analysis. *Psychological Trauma: Theory, Research, Practice, and Policy, 5*(2), 176–183.

Swenson, C. R. (2000). How can we account for DBT's widespread popularity? *Clinical Psychology: Science and Practice, 7*(1), 87–91.

Tummala-Narra, P., Liang, B., & Harvey, M. R. (2007). Aspects of safe attachment in the recovery from trauma. *Journal of Aggression, Maltreatment and Trauma, 14*(3), 1–18.

van der Kolk, B. A., Pelcovitz, D., Roth, S., Mandel, F. S., McFarlane, A., & Herman, J. L. (1996). Dissociation, somatization, and affect dysregulation: The complexity of adaptation to trauma. *American Journal of Psychiatry, 153*(7, Suppl.), 83–93.

van der Kolk, B. A., Roth, S., Pelcovitz, D., Sunday, S., & Spinazzola, J. (2005). Disorders of extreme stress: The empirical foundation of a complex adaptation to trauma. *Journal of Traumatic Stress, 18*(5), 389–399.

Vicarious Trauma Toolkit, The. (n.d.) Retrieved from *https://vtt.ovc.ojp.gov.*

Wagner, A. W., Rizvi, S. L., & Harned, M. S. (2007). Applications of dialectical behavior therapy to the treatment of complex trauma-related problems: When one case formulation does not fit all. *Journal of Traumatic Stress, 20*(4), 391–400.

Yalom, I. D., & Leszcz, M. (2005). *The theory and practice of group psychotherapy* (5th ed.). New York: Perseus Books.

Zanarini, M., Frankenburg, F., Reich, B., Hennen, J., & Silk, K. (2005). Adult experiences of abuse reported by borderline patients and Axis II comparison subjects over six years of prospective follow-up. *Journal of Nervous and Mental Disease, 193*(6), 412–416.

Zanarini, M. C., Williams, A. A., Lewis, R. E., & Reich, R. B. (1997). Reported pathological childhood experiences associated with the development of borderline personality disorder. *American Journal of Psychiatry, 154*(8), 1101.

Zlotnick, C., Shea, M. T., Rosen, K. H., Simpson, E., Mulrenin, K., & Begin, A. (1997). An affect-management group for women with posttraumatic stress disorder and histories of childhood sexual abuse. *Journal of Traumatic Stress, 10,* 425–436.

Index